Keto Diet

The Ultimate Guide to Everything Keto; Includes Recipes and a 7 day Meal Plan

Jane Peters

FREE 25 Ketogenic Diet Dessert Recipes eBook

Download Your **FREE** copy of 25 Ketogenic Diet Dessert Recipes eBook!

Includes Readers Newsletter

Sign up to our newsletter to receive news on new book releases, discounts, and free Kindle book promotions. All books will be available as paperback, audio, on Kindle and Kindle Unlimited unless otherwise stated. We focus on publishing books that can help people in all aspects of life on a variety of topics. Start your learning journey today!

Go to the link below!

http://dibblypublishing.com/free-25ketodessertrecipes/

Follow Us on Social Media

https://www.facebook.com/dibblypublishing/

https://twitter.com/DibblyPublish

For extra content on self-improvement and personal growth visit:

https://masterlifechallenge.com

Table of Contents

Introduction 11

Chapter 1 13

What is A Ketogenic Diet? 13
  Types of Ketogenic Diet 14
  A Basic Breakdown of the Ketogenic Diet 15
  The Body's Natural Process of Energy Production 17
  Changing the Body's Natural Process with the Ketogenic Diet
 18
      Loss of salts 19
      Changes in the bowel habits 19
      Bad breath 20
      Leg Cramps 20
      Loss of Energy 20
      Keto flu 21
  What is Ketosis? 22
  Isn't Ketosis Dangerous? 22
      Ketoacidosis 23
      Blood test 24
      Urine test 25
      Breath test 25
  How Does the Ketogenic Diet Differ From Other Diets? 26
      1. Sustained state of ketosis 26
      2. Addresses weight loss and health conditions. 26
      3. Focuses on the nutrients 26
  Do I Need Medical Supervision on the Ketogenic Diet? 27

Chapter 2 29

Benefits of the Ketogenic Diet 29
      1. The Ketogenic Diet Causes a Reduction in Appetite ...30
      2. No Sudden Drops in Blood Sugar 30
      3. Reduced Blood Pressure 31
      4. Increased HDL Levels 31
      5. Increased Weight Loss 32
      6. Reduced Triglycerides 33
      7. Reduced Cholesterol 33
      8. Reduced Belly Fat 33

9. Reduced Insulin Levels...34
10. Improved Mental Health..35
11. Improved Digestion..35

Chapter 3 ....**37**

Eating Guidelines for the Ketogenic Diet...................................37
Proteins..39
Seafood..40
Fats and Oils 40
Vegetables..42
Dairy...42
Spices and Additives 43
Supplements...43
What to drink..44
What to Avoid **45**

Chapter 4 ....**48**

Ketogenic 7 Day Meal Plan...48
The Ketogenic Meal Plan Guidelines **48**
1. Have a clear guideline on the amount of protein that you
need. 48
2. Set the amount of carbs that you need per day 49
7 Day Ketogenic Diet Meal Plan **50**
Day One 50
Day Two..51
Day three 51
Day Four...52
Day Five..53
Day six 54
Day seven 55

Chapter 5 ....**57**

Ketogenic Breakfast Recipes...57
1. Scrambled Eggs 57
2. Frittata with fresh spinach 58
3. Cereal with Cacao Nibs 59
4. Grain free hemp heart porridge 61
5. Almond Joy Pancakes 63
Instructions 63
6. Bacon and Avocado 64

7.   Green Buttered Eggs 65
8.   Cheddar and Chive Soufflés 67
9.   Swiss Chard and Ricotta Pie 68
10. Egg Fat Breakfast Biscuit...70
11. Avocado and Salmon..71
12. Keto White Pizza Frittata 72

Chapter 6 ....**75**

Ketogenic Lunch Recipes **75**
1.   Chicken Pad Thai 75
2.   Crockpot Chicken Stew..77
3.   Vegan Sesame Tofu and Eggplant...........................78
4.   Salmon Patties with Fresh herbs............................80
5.   Lamb Meatballs with Cauliflower Pilaf.................81
6.   Cheesy Spinach Rolls with Apple Slaw 83
7.   Low Carb Chicken Quesadilla................................85
8.   Chipotle Steak bowl 87
9. Low Carb Garlic Shrimp Pasta 89
10. Green Bean Fries...90
11. Easy Buffalo Wings..92
12. Juicy Butter Burgers 93

Chapter 7 ....**96**

Ketogenic Dinner Recipes...**96**
1.   Lemon Rosemary Chicken with Roasted Broccolini 96
2.   Crockpot Double Beef 97
3.   Roasted Brussels Sprouts with Bacon 98
4.   Roasted Garlic and Rosemary Cauliflower Mash................100
5.   Lemon Garlic Shrimp Kabobs................................101
6.   Low Carb Skillet Brownies 102
7.   Prawn and Chorizo Frittata 104
8.   Cheese and Onion pork chops................................105
9.   Seafood Curry 106
10. Cured Pollock with dill cream and radish salad 108
11. Cloud Bread..111
12. Greek salad omelet...112

Chapter 8 ....**114**

Ketogenic Snacks/Desserts Recipes **114**
1.   Low carb cheesecake 114

2.   Caramel Nut Clusters 116
3.   Low Carb Peanut Butter Cookies............................118
4.   Salted Caramel Custard 119
5.   Walnut Keto Fudge............................120
6.   Coconut Cream with Berries 121
7.   Berries and whipped Cream 122
8.   Pumpkin Pecan Tart............................123
9. Sugar-Free Chocolate Chips 125
10.   Basic Oopsie Rolls 126

Chapter 9 ....**128**
Tips to help you succeed at the Ketogenic Diet............................**128**
1.   Calorie Intake and the Ketogenic Diet 128
2.   Hydration and the Ketogenic Diet............................129
3.   The Ketogenic Diet and Your Budget............................129
4.   Traveling While Eating Keto............................130
5.   Fast Food Choices and Keto............................130
6.   Working out on a Ketogenic Diet 131
7.   Fasting and Ketosis............................131

Conclusion **133**
Don't Forget to Download Your FREE 25 Ketogenic Diet Dessert Recipes............................**134**
Other Books Published by Dibbly Publishing **134**

Introduction

With the numerous challenges that the world seems to face regarding the best diet that can be adopted for continued health, the ketogenic diet has been proven to be one of those diets that help in addressing numerous issues related to healthy living. Most of the diet plans tend to focus more on helping people reduce weight however as you get to understand more about ketogenic diet, you realize that it's not just about losing weight but also experiencing some of the dynamic health benefits that come with the body shifting from utilizing glucose as the primary source of energy to utilizing fats.

After getting an in-depth insight regarding the ketogenic diet, you then will wonder why a majority of the people are shying away from maximizing the numerous benefits associated with being on this diet. This could be due to the fact that many people have grown up hearing a lot of misconceptions regarding diets that are high in fats and hardly take time to verify the kind of fats that should be avoided and why getting on a high-fat diet could be the solution to some of the health conditions that we daily struggle with.

Keto Diet: The Ultimate Guide to Everything Keto, is a book that has shared in-depth insight regarding what the keto diet entails. When you understand what the keto diet is all about and how shifting from a high carbohydrate way of life to a low carb, high fat and medium protein can be of great benefit to you then you will not hesitate to give it a try. All the topics have been delved with in detail which then offers you a clear picture of what the diet is and how it can be implemented for successful results. From understanding the ketogenic diet, the process of ketosis to benefits of the ketogenic diet, you will be able to get helpful insight regarding the diet that you can immediately take advantage of.

A Ketogenic diet has been proven to be helpful in diverse ways which range from prevention of health conditions like heart attack, diabetes and stroke, diseases that majorly thrive when you are on a high carbohydrate diet. Cases of poor mental health like depression, unhealthy eating habits, and other addictions can be effectively addressed by adopting a ketogenic diet which is mainly a low carb, moderate protein, and high-fat diet. Following strict diet guidelines have been a major challenge for many people who intend to realize the health benefits associated with such diets, and in many cases, most people fall off because of the intense guidelines of having to measure calories or even choose the type of foods to eat like in most diet plans.

The Ketogenic diet is a very flexible form of diet as you don't have to choose foods every time you intend to eat something, even measuring calories is not important. All that you have to focus on is to ensure that your food intake per day is according to the stated ratios of about 5% carbohydrates, 20% protein and 75% fats. Once you have adapted to the process of ketosis, then you will immediately begin to realize the benefits associated with the diet. Benefits like improved mental efficiency and weight loss are just a few of what you get to experience after being on the keto diet just for a few weeks.

Take your time and go through the entire book as each topic has valuable information that you can immediately take advantage of in your dieting journey.

Also, please don't forget to download your free copy of **25 Ketogenic Dessert Recipes** to supplement all the other recipes you will find in the last chapters.

Chapter 1

What is A Ketogenic Diet?

A ketogenic diet, also known as low carb high-fat diet or keto diet, is a high fat, medium protein, and low carbohydrate diet. It entails production of ketones by the liver which then shifts the body's metabolism to utilizing fat as a source of energy instead of glucose. A person who is on a ketogenic diet gets into a metabolic state known as ketosis and while in that state, the body utilizes ketone bodies for energy instead of glucose. Ketone bodies are derived from consumption of high fats and have been proven to provide a steady supply of energy, unlike glucose that's derived from intake of carbohydrates.

Ketogenic diets work more like other diets where the intake of calories is limited putting the body into a state of caloric deficit. When the body is in such a state, it then gets to burn more energy than what's consumed. There are numerous benefits that have been associated with being on a ketogenic diet and, apart from being a great tool for weight loss, it also helps in reducing the risks of health conditions like diabetes, stroke, heart diseases, epilepsy, Alzheimer's and more. One thing that distinguishes a ketogenic diet from other forms of dieting is the fact that it doesn't work in phases, once you switch to a ketogenic diet, you are expected to sustain intake of the low carb, moderate protein, and high fat consistently until your body switches and adapts to ketosis.

The macronutrient ratios in a ketogenic diet consist of high fat between 60 – 80%, moderate protein between 15 – 35% and low carbohydrate of 5%. Eating according to the stated ratios helps in depleting the body of glucose which then forces it to start the production of ketones. The body then automatically switches to use of ketones for energy. Achieving that state of ketosis takes effort, especially for beginners that are shifting to a ketogenic diet. This is mainly because most of the common foods that you get to consume have high levels of carbohydrates and it, therefore, takes a concerted effort to be able to restrict the intake of carbohydrates to achieve that shift by the body to ketosis.

Types of Ketogenic Diet

There are various ways through which the body can be brought into the state of ketosis. It is important that you choose the type that best suits your ideal needs given some people engage in intensive activities that require more energy.

Below are some of the types of ketogenic diet:

Standard ketogenic diet: This is one of the common types of ketogenic diet that most people follow. The diet consists of consuming minimal carbohydrates alongside a moderate protein and very high fats. The meals are eaten in the ratio of carbs 5%, Protein 20% or less, and fats can be 75% or more. Regarding measurement of grams per day, carbohydrates would be between 20 – 50g, protein would be between 60 – 80g while there is no limit to the amount of fat you can take as it's what enables the body to generate energy.

Targeted Ketogenic diet: This type of diet requires an intake of the food ratios as indicated in the standard diet. However, the individual gets to incorporate carbs that get digested fast before commencing your exercise routine. The diet is ideal for those engaging in tough activities that require a lot of energy. Consume 25 – 50 net carbs 30 minutes before your workout. The intent is to provide a boost of energy for your workouts. The carbs should be burned efficiently and shouldn't disrupt your ketosis. Your post-workout meal should be high in protein for muscle recovery and nutrient absorption.

Cyclical ketogenic diet: This type of ketogenic diet requires being on the standard ketogenic diet for about five days then alternating with one or two days of eating high carb foods, about 400 – 600 grams of carbs. This form of diet is suitable for those who are involved in activities that require high energy levels, mainly used by body builders and athletes to maximize fat loss while building lean muscle mass.

High Protein ketogenic diet: The type of ketogenic diet is quite similar to the standard although there is a difference in the high quantity of protein that one gets to consume. The ration for high protein ketogenic diet may include carbs at 5% or less, protein 35% or more and fat at 60%.

A Basic Breakdown of the Ketogenic Diet

Successful keto dieting involves balancing macronutrient ratios with the intake of carbohydrates being limited to about 50 grams per day or less. When you are starting out on the ketogenic diet, it's advisable that the intake of carbohydrates be limited to about 20 grams or less to enable the body to get into ketosis. As you become strict with your dieting at the initial stages, it then becomes much easier for your body to enter into ketosis. Ensure that you track accurately the macronutrients of the foods that you consume so that the condition of ketosis is sustained.

There are recommended ratios for the protein, carbohydrates, and fats to be consumed. However, the exact amount can be decided depending on your activity levels and body response. One of the reasons that motivates many people to be on a ketogenic diet is the ability to lose weight relatively fast. Consuming foods that have high-calorie levels leads to excess weight, being on a low carb diet reduces the intake of calories which results in weight loss. When you are on a ketogenic diet, your body tends to burn more calories as your body gets to operate on fat metabolism. Eating a diet that's high in fat also makes you feel more satisfied.

Being on a ketogenic diet impacts the blood sugar levels effectively and with stable blood sugar levels, the false hunger pains and food cravings are reduced drastically.

Consumption of foods high in carbohydrates causes the levels of blood glucose to rise quite fast, and that can contribute to a rapid release of insulin by the pancreatic glands to help stabilize the blood sugar levels. Insulin is a hormone that signals your body to store fat, and when insulin levels are high, it may result in a metabolic syndrome leading to constant hunger feelings, weight gain and other issues. Reduction of insulin levels in your body is therefore essential for the success of any diet. When the level of insulin in your body is kept low, then an environment is created that limits storage of fats while at the same time promoting fat lipolysis.

Being on a ketogenic diet also makes you eat more nutritious foods and less processed foods. Most people have the belief that eating a lot of fat is bad but various studies have proved that eating monounsaturated and saturated fats do not expose you to the risks of getting heart disease.

The Body's Natural Process of Energy Production

Being on a diet that's high in carbohydrates makes the body burn glucose for fuel and can store up to 2000 calories as glucose energy. The body finds it easy to utilize glucose as a source of energy and will often choose glucose over any other source of energy. When there is excess glucose in the body, it raises insulin which then drives the excess glucose to be stored as glycogen in the skeletal cells. Insulin also drives the excess glucose into the fat cells for storage as fats. It also helps with the processing of glucose into the blood stream, and since glucose is the primary source of energy being utilized by the body, fats are therefore not used, so they end up being stored.

If you reduce the intake of carbohydrates and replace it with high fat and moderate protein, the level of insulin also drops since there is less glucose. With insulin levels being low, the liver gets to burn fat for fuel. It's normally impossible for your body to automatically burn the stored fat for fuel when insulin in the body is high. The burning of fat by your body results in the production of ketones which are fatty acids that can be utilized directly by body cells, the heart, the brain and other body organs. So, lowering the intake of carbohydrates, therefore, induces your body into a state of ketosis, a natural state that gets initiated whenever your body is running low on glucose or starvation.

The fact that your body is utilizing fat for fuel is not a guarantee that it has adapted to the process as it takes a few days or even over a week for your body to fully adapt to ketosis. When the stored energy gets depleted, your body then gets to lose energy which then creates a demand for sugar, and such a feeling can be quite tempting for you to resort to easier ways of replenishing the depleted energy. Your body has, over time, built a combination of enzymes that handle the process with only a few dealings with fats. So, as you reduce the intake of carbohydrates, your body gets an increase in fat levels which causes new enzymes that can process the fats to be released. As your body begins to adapt to a ketosis state it then utilizes all the glucose that could still be in your system which means all the glycogen that could still be in the muscles gets depleted.

Such an occurrence may lead to a lack of energy in the body and feelings of lethargy. A person transitioning from a traditional diet to a ketogenic diet may, in the first week, experience feelings of mental fogginess, headaches, dizziness, flue like symptoms and aggravation.

It's advisable that you increase intake of sodium at this stage as it helps with the replenishing of the electrolytes while enhancing water retention. It takes about two weeks to effectively adapt to a ketogenic diet and cutting the intake of carbohydrates to about 5 grams, as it helps in ensuring you get to a state of ketosis sooner.

Changing the Body's Natural Process with the Ketogenic Diet

Once the body adapts to ketosis, it then gets to utilize fats as the primary source of energy. Eating foods which are high in fats with moderate protein and low carbs can have such a massive impact on your health such as lowering levels of cholesterol, blood sugar, body weight, and raising energy levels. The significant change in the diet can also cause some of the side effects as your body gets to adapt to the changes. However, most of the side effects are temporary and can be addressed.

- Some of the side effects may include the following:

- Loss of salts

- Changes in the bowel habits

- Bad breath

- Leg cramps

- Loss of energy

- Keto flu

Loss of salts

Being on a ketogenic diet also increases the ability for the kidney to remove salts from the blood. The changes in the balance of fluids, in your body, takes place when your body utilizes the stored glycogen, leading to a release of water in the form of urine. This process depletes the salts in your body, so it's important that you increase the intake of salt. Failure to raise intake of sodium may cause all the symptoms associated with electrolyte deficiency like nausea, trouble with sleeping and others. To address the situation, ensure that you're hydrated throughout the day by increasing your intake of water.

Ensuring you consume enough sodium is key to reducing your chances of side effects. Other minerals like potassium and magnesium are also important and can be taken as supplements.

Changes in the bowel habits

Shifting to a ketogenic diet may also come with changes in your bowel movements such as experiencing constipation. Your bowel habits should, however, improve within a short time, especially if you're consuming enough fiber. To address the situation, you can consider consuming nonstarchy foods like legumes, fibrous vegetables, nuts, and seeds.

Bad breath

Bad breath can occur when you are entering the fat burning state of ketosis. Ketones are released through the urine, sweat, and breath and there is a component of ketone known as acetone, which when released, creates a metallic taste in your mouth and the smell is not very pleasant. Bad breath, however, only lasts for a few days and then disappears after your body has adapted to ketosis. If you find bad breath to be disturbing, you can use breath freshener or sugar-free mint to address the situation. You can also consider having enhanced oral hygiene by either using mouth wash or brushing your teeth more frequently.

Leg Cramps

Muscle cramps are a common side effect that has been associated with a ketogenic diet and typically occurs when there is a loss of minerals in the blood, especially sodium. Leg cramps can be avoided by drinking plenty of water and an increase in sodium consumption. You may also consider the use of supplements to help with boosting your level of minerals in your body.

Loss of Energy

Due to the reduction of carbohydrate consumption, you will notice that it takes time for your body to adapt given it has been using carbohydrates as its main fuel source. Such a shift may lead to loss of energy, but it only lasts for a short period. To address the situation, you can avoid activities that require the use of a lot of energy, like engaging in intensive exercises. Remember, consuming carbohydrates while in such a state may further delay your progress with the ketogenic diet.

As your body adjusts to burning fat for energy, there will be feelings of dehydration and lack of salt due to frequent urination. So, the best thing to do is to drink plenty of water and electrolytes to make it easier for your body to transition well without resorting to eating foods that may jeopardize the process.

Keto flu

This is a common side effect of being on a ketogenic diet, although it only takes place for a few days as you start off. Keto flu is a way your body reacts to carb withdrawal and mainly a result of your body shifting from the normal way of operation to ketosis. This is the time when your body has not yet fully adapted to the process of ketosis as the cells, and the organs are beginning to demand ketones. You will start to experience these symptoms by the end of your first week on a ketogenic diet, in some cases earlier. The symptoms include; brain fogginess or slow thinking, fatigue, dizziness, faster heart beat especially when lying down, cravings and insomnia, amongst others. This is the first phase of fat adaptation, and once you get through this first step, you will begin to feel better.

The best way of addressing the side effect is by allowing your body to adapt to the process quickly. This adaptation can be made by lowering the intake of carbohydrates over a number of weeks. Reduce the intake of carbohydrates in a gradual way instead of shifting suddenly to a low consumption of carbs. Remember, intake of salt and water helps keep you hydrated. If you find yourself struggling with the side effects then instead of falling off the ketogenic diet, you can adjust the intake of carbohydrates slightly. Increase carbohydrate consumption as a last resort. You should also ensure that you consume a sufficient amount of fat. After you get through the carb withdrawal process, you are more likely to experience weight loss, although, there are people who hardly experience withdrawal effects.

What is Ketosis?

Ketosis can be defined as a metabolic state where the liver gets to break down fats stored in the body as a source of fuel. It is a nutritional process which takes place when the body lacks carbohydrates in the cells needed for energy. The body then automatically shifts to burning fat for fuel. The byproduct produced through the process is known as ketones which are then used by the body as energy. The three types of ketone bodies are; acetone, beta-hydroxybutyrate and acetoacetate acid. Most of the body cells can directly utilize the ketones as a source of energy in a far better way than they use glucose.

Although most of the cells in the body can effectively use the produced ketones, there are specific cells in the body that still require glucose like the red cells, parts of the brain and the cells in the eyes. The good thing is that the liver is well equipped with sufficient enzymes that help in producing glucose from the consumed protein through a process known as gluconeogenesis. The liver then creates the new sugar as required by those vital organs. Ketosis has been proven to be quite healthy as it helps with improving health conditions, especially in situations where you have conditions like; diabetes, cardiovascular disease, and metabolic syndrome. It's also been proven that being in a state of ketosis helps with improving the levels of good cholesterol compared to carbohydrates.

Isn't Ketosis Dangerous?

Even as the keto diet continues to rise in popularity, with many people preferring over other diets, many people still shy away from the keto diet due to a condition known as ketoacidosis. Ketosis is not dangerous, and that's a fact that has been proven many times. However, a person with various illnesses like, diabetes type 1, should seek the advice of a doctor before starting a keto diet.

Ketoacidosis

Ketoacidosis is a condition that arises when the level of ketones in the body is overproduced which then makes the body highly acidic. It's one of the risks that have been associated with ketosis and happens amongst those with type 1 diabetes or other illnesses that trigger production of hormones that work against insulin in the body. Some of the common triggers of this condition include; emotional trauma, drug abuse, stress, physical trauma, and surgery. A person who has a proper functioning pancreas may not experience ketoacidosis.

The condition can be tested easily at home by using kits, especially when you notice that there are increased levels of ketones in the urine alongside high levels of blood sugar. Some of the common symptoms that can be associated with ketoacidosis include;

- Abdominal pains

- Lack of proper concentration or even confusion

- Dry skin

- Dry mouth and excessive thirst

- Nausea and vomiting

- Rapid breathing and shortness of breath.

For those who have type 1 diabetes; the following measures can be immediately taken to address the situation.

- Get your body rehydrated by consuming a lot of water to dilute the excess sugar that could be in your system.

- Electrolyte replacement can also be done so that your body's cells, muscles, and the nerves are kept healthy and functioning.

- Insulin therapy can also be undertaken to reverse the condition.

To address the situation and keep it from occurring; the level of ketone in your body should be consistently ascertained for perfect health. If you have type 1 diabetes, then do not start a ketogenic diet without seeking your Doctor's advice. For accurate test results, you can use breath meter instead of the strips as the strips only measure ketones that have been wasted. Below are some of the ways you can test for ketones:

Blood test

This test can be carried to ascertain the level of ketones in the blood. A glucose meter can be used to conduct the tests. This test is one of the most effective ones and the best way to ascertain whether the body is well adapted to the ketosis process. When the body is well adapted to ketosis, the levels of blood sugar are mostly in a balanced state of about 50 – 75 mg/dl. When you are in this state, you will feel quite good and with a lot of stamina and mental strength. The overall mood and behavior will also be great. It's a good sign that your body has effectively embraced the use of ketones as a source of energy and is not anymore dependent on carbs. Your body is therefore relaxed and not struggling with keeping the blood sugar levels at a healthy state.

Urine test

This test entails checking the urine for the level of ketones and can be done using a urine strip. This is one of the ways of knowing the level of acetone in the urine although, some of the tests may not be as accurate. Urine ketone strips are cheap and some most commonly used compared to other methods of measuring ketone levels. One reason that makes the test inaccurate is the fact that the body, in the initial phase, tends to release a lot of ketones before actually adapting to the process. Once the body adjusts to the process, the level of ketones released is reduced. If the amount of ketones remains high, even after adapting to ketosis, then that could be an indicator that the body cells may be having problems.

The changes in hydration are also likely to alter the levels of ketone concentration. If you are well hydrated, then the amount of ketones in the urine will be more diluted.

Breath test

A breath meter is what can be used to test for ketone levels in your breath. It's a more cost-effective method of testing the level of acetone in the body. However, the breath ketones may not accurately express the level of ketones in the blood. A breath test is one that has been proven to be quite accurate, and the device used for carrying out the test can be bought once and be utilized only when required. The device is not complicated and can be easily used by breathing through the mouth piece showing the unique colors based on the level of ketones in the body.

For accurate results, you can opt for the blood test as it has the highest accuracy rating.

How Does the Ketogenic Diet Differ From Other Diets?

Below are some of the factors that distinguish the ketogenic diet from other forms of dieting:

1. Sustained state of ketosis

One thing that distinguishes a ketogenic diet from other types of dieting is the fact that the ketogenic diet gets you into a continuous nutritional state known as ketosis. Although most low carb diets can equally get you into that state, it's not at a sustained level. For example, paleo diet recommends the intake of whole foods and not processed foods and grains. Although you can experience a state of ketosis while on Paleo diet, it's not sustained as consumption of foods that are rich in starch, like potatoes, can quickly put you out of ketosis.

2. Addresses weight loss and health conditions.

Another thing that distinguishes a ketogenic diet from other types of diets are the numerous benefits that one gets to enjoy while on a ketogenic diet. You don't just get to experience weight loss; it can also be a solution to numerous health conditions like heart problems, diabetes, epilepsy and much more.

3. Focuses on the nutrients

Unlike Paleo diet or other diets, ketogenic diet focuses mostly on the carbs, proteins, and fats where success with the diet majorly depends on the ratios of the macronutrients consumed. Other diets like Paleo mostly focuses on food choices where one gets to eliminate grains, processed foods, and dairy and is also free to balance the food choices as desired.

Some additional factors that distinguish a ketogenic diet from other forms of dieting include:

- Long-term weight loss

- Reduced levels of blood pressure

- Reduced levels of craving

- Enhanced levels of satiety

- Increased resistance to insulin.

- Reduced cases of inflammation

- Reduced risks of getting heart disease, amongst others.

Do I Need Medical Supervision on the Ketogenic Diet?

Just as we shared earlier, it's advisable that you consult with a medical supervisor if you have medical conditions that could endanger your life before starting a ketogenic diet. Some of the conditions associated with being on a ketogenic diet, like ketoacidosis, arise as a result of you adopting the diet without getting proper advice from your doctor. Before you start a ketogenic diet, ensure that you carry out complete blood profile where you can ascertain the conditions of the following:

- Liver function

- Insulin

- Vitamin D

Remember, the fact that you experience resistance as you start doesn't necessarily mean that the diet is not ideal for you. Mostly, resistance arises as a result of cholesterol phobia or fat phobia, but it only lasts for a short period.

Chapter 2

Benefits of the Ketogenic Diet

There are many advantages that can be associated with the ketogenic diet, and the effectiveness of the diet begins with the metabolic process of ketosis and the impact it can have on the numerous cells within the body. When the body cells are healthy and work efficiently, it also impacts the wellbeing of an individual, and that's something that's enhanced when you are on a ketogenic diet. Eating foods with high level of carbohydrates often lead to cell damage, resulting in numerous health conditions. The foods tend to increase the amount of insulin and glucose in the blood stream and, as much as glucose is great for energy, having it in excess has the potential of harming the body systems.

Although it's difficult to know how much can be too much, let's look at this example. A healthy individual has been said to have dissolved sugar in the blood stream of about a teaspoon, but in most cases, you realize that a can of soft drink alone has about ten teaspoons. When broken down, it can result into about 16 teaspoons of sugar getting into the blood stream. High carbohydrate foods provide excess glucose that the body can hardly handle. Blood glucose is liquid sugar, and just as it looks sticky when spilled in your hands, it's equally sticky while in your body. The stickiness results into a condition known as glycation.

Glycation is a process where excess blood sugar sticks and begins to damage the body tissues and proteins. The injured body tissues then fail to function effectively which causes a chain of events that lead to inflammation. The inflammatory conditions can be effectively repressed by the presence of ketones in the cells. Ketones help with enhancing the health and efficiency of cells while also reducing oxidative stress in the body. The more fat you burn for fuel, instead of carbohydrates, the better and healthier you become.

Below are some of the benefits that can be associated with a ketogenic diet:

1. The Ketogenic Diet Causes a Reduction in Appetite

One of the most outstanding benefits of being on a ketogenic diet is the ability to reduce appetite. When your appetite is not reduced, you will have cravings for carb filled foods. Overcoming the temptation to eat then becomes quite difficult. When you shift from a high carbohydrate diet to a high-fat diet, you then begin to stop experiencing swings in blood sugar levels. The fluctuations in blood sugar levels are what is attributed to intense cravings for carbohydrates. Therefore, by being on a high-fat diet, the ketones produced suppresses your appetite as it also frees you from sugar cravings that may lead to consumption of junk food. More subtly, ketones have the potential of controlling the hormones responsible for hunger and satiation as fat is a more satisfying source of energy.

2. No Sudden Drops in Blood Sugar

Foods that are high in carbohydrates gets metabolized much faster although, the energy gets depleted quickly, forcing you to eat a snack or a meal to sustain energy levels. When you are on a ketogenic diet, you are more likely to overcome sudden drops of blood sugar levels as the state of ketosis ensures that your body has sufficient amount of energy. The blood sugar levels, therefore, get to normalize as there are no drastic shifts in the level of energy.

3. Reduced Blood Pressure

Being on a ketogenic diet helps with stabilizing the blood sugar levels as carbohydrates are the primary macronutrient that raises your blood sugar. A high carb diet raises the levels of blood sugar as the pancreas is prompted for insulin release to handle excess glucose. In case you are on medication, it's advisable that you consult with your doctor so that you don't continue with both the diet and the medication at the same time.

4. Increased HDL Levels

There is a common misconception about high-fat diets that they have the potential of increasing cholesterol levels in the body which then ends up clogging the arteries. Low carb diets are known to improve metabolism rates and have been proven to optimize the levels of cholesterol while also improving heart health. HDL cholesterol is mostly known as the good cholesterol and works by collecting cholesterol that is not used through the body cells by bringing them back to the liver for recycling. This action helps in preventing cholesterol from accumulating around the arteries which may lead to the clogging of the arteries.

Being on a ketogenic diet enhances the production of HDL cholesterol, the more fat you eat, the higher the HDL cholesterol becomes which is a good thing. HDL cholesterol has anti-inflammatory effects which help in reducing cases of inflammation while lowering the risk of cardio vascular conditions.

5. Increased Weight Loss

The ability to realize a rapid weight loss is one of the most attractive benefits associated with the ketogenic diet. By strictly lowering the intake of carbohydrates, the body utilizes most of the fats without having to store more which greatly improves muscle mass. When on a ketogenic diet, your appetite gets suppressed reducing cravings for foods that are more likely to spur weight gain. By altering the concentration of hormones responsible for hunger, you can easily go for a longer period without feeling hungry resulting in weight loss. To effectively use a ketogenic diet for weight loss, you should ensure that you consider the following:

- Ensure that your diet consists of high fats between 70 – 80% in the form of calories.

- Ensure that you moderate the intake of proteins between 20 – 25% of total calories.

- The low carbohydrates concentration should be 5%, and, in some cases, no more than 10%.

Numbers may vary depending on your height, weight, lean body mass and gender, amongst other things. Maintaining a healthy weight is much easier while on a keto diet as you feel satiated most of the time.

6.   Reduced Triglycerides

Triglycerides are a type of dietary fat that's mostly found in cooking oils, meats and dairy products and can either be converted to energy for use by the body or be stored as fat. When you consume food, the body converts the excess calories that you are not immediately utilizing into triglycerides which are then stored in the cells for later use. If your diet consists of high carbohydrates, then there are chances that you have high amounts of triglycerides.

Consumption of carbohydrates does, in a great way, contribute to the increased levels of triglycerides. As you shift to a ketogenic diet, the levels of triglycerides come down which contributes to reduced chances of contracting various ailments.

7. Reduced Cholesterol

High carb foods can significantly increase the levels of cholesterol increasing your chances of stroke or heart disease. There are two types of cholesterol, the low-density lipoprotein (LDL), the bad cholesterol, causing fats to build up around the arteries. The other type is high-density lipoprotein (HDL), known as the good cholesterol, enabling the body to get rid of the excess cholesterol.

The ketogenic diet helps in reducing the level of bad cholesterol in the body resulting in a reduced risk of heart disease and other ailments.

8. Reduced Belly Fat

As much as you can have fat on different parts of the body, belly fat is a kind of fat that doesn't just sit still as it's more likely to overlap and cover other areas, especially your abs. Eliminating belly fat can be challenging and reducing the intake of carbohydrates helps in reducing belly fat. The keto diet's appetite suppression helps the regulation of your body functions and normalizes weight. Combining keto diet with exercises can greatly reduce your body fat, resulting in well-toned muscles.

To effectively lose stubborn belly fat through ketosis, you can engage in the following:

- Ensure that you hydrate yourself effectively. You can also add broth from bones and vegetables into your meals.

- Include high-intensity work outs to enhance the fat burning effect.

- You can limit the intake of carbohydrates to about 10% of all your daily food calories. You may also increase intake of fats and maintain healthy levels of protein in your diet.

- Remember, sufficient sleep is equally vital as less sleep may cause stress hormones to be triggered and that can jeopardize the process of losing weight.

9. Reduced Insulin Levels

Being on a ketogenic diet can be quite helpful in reducing the amount of insulin that gets released by the pancreas. Reducing the intake of carbohydrates can substantially reduce insulin levels, and that's what a well formulated ketogenic diet is capable of. Being on a ketogenic diet makes you lose any form of cravings for sugar or starch that would otherwise exist. Being in a ketosis state also activates leptin, a hormone that signals the brain when you are satisfied helping reduce blood sugar and insulin levels to normal.

10. Improved Mental Health

Today's traditional way of eating, high carbohydrates, has been linked to causing increase in conditions like diabetes, obesity and other mental disorders like eating disorder, anxiety, and depression. The constant snacking culture of the modern society has a way of negatively impacting the health of your brain. Although, weight loss is such a major benefit when on a ketogenic diet, the improved functioning of the brain is also a benefit that's quite major. Being on this diet has the potential of enhancing brain functionality, like memory retention and so forth, as it's been proven just like heart performance tends to improve, the brain equally improves efficiency while on a keto diet. Therefore, burning fat for energy, instead of glucose, greatly enhances the neuro-therapeutic and neuro-protective capabilities.

The cognitive performance and mental acuity of the brain also get to improve when the brain is operating on ketones, given their soluble nature and ability to effectively feed the brain. Mental health is one of the primary benefits that you get to experience when you are on a ketogenic diet.

11. Improved Digestion

Good health is known to begin with a healthy gut, and over 70% of the immune system is in the gut so being on a diet that's high in carbohydrates releases things like sugar, additives, antibiotics, and pesticides that end up affecting the good bacteria that are required in the intestinal tract. By shifting to a ketogenic diet, it helps in producing more of the good bacteria while also eliminating the bad bacteria which helps in improving the digestion process.

In summary, if you are interested in a diet that can help you realize the below benefits then it's worth giving the ketogenic diet a try:

- Ability to stay full during most times of the day

- Ability to enjoy improved energy levels.

- Ability to overcome addiction to eating patterns that are unhealthy

- Ability to live a healthy life and be able to overcome the diseases that are associated with being overweight.

- Reduced risks of getting certain chronic diseases.

- Improved health and slowed aging process

- Steady weight loss that can be sustained for a longer period.

Chapter 3
Eating Guidelines for the Ketogenic Diet

The eating guidelines for ketogenic diet provide a clear insight on how the diet can be implemented to realize success. Some of the things that should be looked out for when planning on a successful implementation of a ketogenic diet are the following:

Monitor intake of carbohydrates: Most people starting a ketogenic diet tend to put more emphasis on the net carbohydrates, and that may not bring the desired results. The focus should be given to ensuring that you eat no more than 20 grams of carbohydrates per day.

Monitor intake of protein: Intake of protein should equally be controlled and restricted to a specific amount as it has the potential of neutralizing the impact of ketosis. You can limit your consumption to about 0.8 grams per pound for those with a lean body mass. Ensuring that you restrict yourself to such a measurement helps in ensuring that you realize success with a ketogenic diet.

Stop having a fat phobia: Success with a ketogenic diet requires consumption of foods that are high in fats. When on a ketogenic diet, fat is the main source of energy, and it's important that you consume it without having any fears. As much as there are many misconceptions surrounding the consumption of high-fat foods, it's important to realize that without consuming the fat, getting into ketosis may be quite a challenge. Following the below guidelines will be helpful to realize success as you go through the process of ketosis adaptation:

- Start off with a clear eating plan in place, and you can plan your meals in a way that enables you to take longer periods of time before eating. Eating after six hours is, however, not recommended.

- The foods that you eat should be according to the required ratio and should be rich in fats with moderate protein and low carbs. Consider including foods like fish, poultry, eggs, red meat, shellfish, and vegetables.

- Even as you plan your measure for carbohydrates, ensure that the ratio is maintained at below 20g per day, up to 50g when starting out. The carbohydrates that you eat should mainly come from vegetables.

- Remember, intake of starchy foods, and some dairy foods can negatively impact the process of ketosis.

- Avoid foods rich in both proteins and carbohydrates, like legumes, especially in the beginning.

- There are foods that are not allowed to be consumed while on a ketogenic diet like foods that have high levels of natural or added sugar. Such foods may include fruits, dried fruits, candies, fruit juices, chocolate and more.

- Unlike other forms of dieting, where you get to choose the kind of foods to eat, the ketogenic diet gives you the freedom to choose foods based on appetite and what you feel comfortable with provided you follow the required ratio. Try to eat foods that enable you to feel satisfied.

- Ensure that you ascertain the carbohydrate counts in the foods that you purchase by checking the labels. Assuming that the foods are low in carbs can lead to intake of high carbohydrates without knowing.

- Consumption of sweetened drinks like sodas or fruit juices is not encouraged as the sugar element is likely to interfere with the ketosis process. Sometimes, words like sugar-free or sugarless can be appealing, but it's important that you take time and look out for the level of carbohydrates in whatever drink or food you're consuming.

Proteins

Proteins are known as the basic building block of a life that's healthy and vibrant. Proteins also help by providing the required chemical reactions that generally occurs within your body. Below are some of the sources of proteins that you should consider eating while on a ketogenic diet:

Although there are numerous foods that are rich in protein; meat and poultry can be considered some of the staple foods that you can eat while on a ketogenic diet. Meat and poultry are rich in various essential vitamins and minerals like potassium, zinc, and selenium. They are also ideal sources of quality protein that helps in the building and preservation of the muscle which gets developed when on a ketogenic diet.

When choosing the type of meat to purchase, it's advisable that you settle for the grass-fed meat instead of others given that such meats are high in omega three fatty acids. Meat and poultry are also good as they do not have any form of carbohydrates. Consumption of eggs is equally important when on a ketogenic. Eggs contain a great combination of your macronutrients necessary for ketosis, and they are very healthy for you.

Seafood

Fish and seafood are good sources of omega three fatty acids which are vital when you are on a ketogenic diet. The health benefits that can be derived from the fatty acids are numerous with a variety of fish, like salmon and shellfish, being rich in vitamin B, potassium and selenium. There is some seafood that contains higher amounts of carbohydrates. Ensure that you consider the amount of carbohydrates that you may be consuming so that you remain within the recommended range.

Seafood that is rich in omega three fatty acids are species like sardines, salmon, and mackerel amongst others. Omega 3 fatty acids help with lowering insulin levels while increasing the sensitivity of insulin in those who are overweight. Omega 3 fatty acids are also known to play an integral part in improving mental health. The majority of the seafood, unlike other forms of fish, are free of carbohydrates, a fact that makes them quite suitable for consumption while on a ketogenic diet.

Fats and Oils

Fats are a great source of energy, in particular for those intending to realize success with a ketogenic diet. Oils are a great source of the fatty acids. Healthy fats can be derived from foods like sunflower oil, olive oil, butter, cream cheese, etc. These oils are known to have unique properties that make their consumption crucial for a person on a ketogenic diet. The oils help in improving the ketone levels while also promoting a sustained level of ketosis.

Consumption of fats, like olive oil, enhances the functionality of the heart given the high level of monounsaturated fat contained in it, making it suitable for reducing your chances of heart disease and related illnesses. Olive oil is pure and does not have any carbohydrate elements in it. Olive oil is also ideal for use while cooking on low heat and salad dressing. Cream and butter are equally good fats that are delicious and worth including in a ketogenic diet since both are free of carbs. There are different types of fats that you may consider consuming like;

Saturated fats: This category includes healthy fats that can be eaten, like ghee, butter, lard and coconut oil.

Monounsaturated fats: This category also contains fats that are suitable while on a ketogenic diet and include avocado, olive oil, and macadamia nut oil.

Polyunsaturated fats: Polyunsaturated fats are also suitable for consumption and are mainly found in fatty fish and animal protein. The processed polyunsaturated fats are, however, not healthy for consumption.

Tran's fats: These are fats that have been altered through a chemical process like hydrogenation, and they may not be very suitable for use while on a ketogenic diet. Some of the trans or processed fats have been linked to being a cause of heart disease.

The monounsaturated and saturated fats have been proven to be more stable chemically and less inflammatory. Since a ketogenic diet emphasizes on a high intake of fats, you can look for various ways on how you can consume the fat for better use by your body.

Vegetables

Consumption of vegetables is vital for anybody on a ketogenic diet as they are non-starchy with low levels of carbohydrates. Vegetables are rich in various nutrients. Fruits and vegetables are good sources of fiber which is not absorbed and digested by the body. Vegetables have low levels of carbohydrates apart from the ones that are starchy, which should be avoided. They are also good antioxidants that protect from free radicals while protecting cell damage. Some of the common types of vegetables that can be consumed include cauliflower, kale, broccoli, etc. These kinds of vegetables help with reduction of conditions like cancer or heart disease.

Dairy

Most of the dairy products are suitable for consumption when on a ketogenic diet, however, emphasis should be given to consuming full-fat dairy items. Like the harder cheeses, which have very low levels of carbohydrates.

Nuts and Seeds

Nuts and seeds are known to have high levels of fats while also low in carbohydrates. Consumption of seeds and nuts helps with the reduction of risks associated with heart disease, depression, cancer, and other chronic ailments. Nuts are good sources of fiber which also helps with enhancing the body's health while at the same time increasing levels of satiation. Common seeds and nuts that you can consider consuming include almonds, macadamia nuts, cashews, pumpkin seeds, sesame seeds, pecans, walnuts, etc.

Spices and Additives

There are various varieties of spices and additives that are available in the market, and the preparation process is what determines what to go for and what should be avoided. When purchasing spices and additives, it's advisable that you go for pure herbs and spices. You can try and prevent the use of additives and spices that are made of unhealthy oils. Avoid those that contain sugars and those labeled as low fat.

Supplements

There are some low carb diet supplements that can be used when on a ketogenic diet. Some of the supplements include the following:

Sodium: When you shift to a ketogenic diet the body gets to lose storage of carbohydrates and in the process, releases a lot of sodium and water. This experience then leads to a drop-in blood sugar levels and results in feelings of tiredness and sluggishness. Intake of additional sodium can significantly help with addressing this situation and should be encouraged during this adaptation process.

Branched chain amino acids: This supplement is suitable for intake after engaging in exercise or some intense activity. The supplement helps in decreasing the damage of tissues that may have come as a result of intensive training. They also help with enhancing the levels of amino acids in the body that are responsible for igniting happiness even during intense exercises.

Whole amino acids: Helps with muscle repair and the recovery process that you experience after an intensive work out. In case of mental stress due to a tough work out, these types of amino acids still allows the body to continue with the hard work instead of shutting down and giving up.

Glutamine: Glutamine supplements help with carbohydrate storage and synthesis of muscle glycogen. They also enhance the production of glucose during exercise.

Taurine: Has a carbohydrate sparing effect and enhances efficient utilization of carbohydrates within the body especially during prolonged exercise. The supplements can be taken before engaging in a tough exercise.

Magnesium: Just like sodium, magnesium equally gets depleted as you switch from a high carb to a low carb diet. Lack of magnesium may lead to things like muscle twitching as a majority of enzymes require magnesium to function effectively.

What to drink

It's important that you stay hydrated while on a ketogenic diet, especially when you are in the adaptation process. However, not all drinks are permitted while on a ketogenic diet, there are some that should be avoided and others embraced. Some of the drinks that are sugar-free and carb free include:

- Diet tonic water

- Liquid water enhancer

- Sugar-free carbonated water

- Sugar-free diet drinks

- Seltzer water

If you love alcohol then you can consider the following as they are both sugar and carb free:

- Tequila

- Whiskey, scotch

- Vodka

- Brandy

- Cognac

- Gin

What to Avoid

Some of the foods that you can avoid when on ketogenic diet include:

Packaged and processed foods: These are foods that have either been processed using some of the chemicals or unhealthy oils that we mentioned earlier. Manufactures are also known to add a lot of preservatives, extra sugar and trans fats to some of these processed foods which make them unhealthy for consumption. Most of these foods have been labeled as low carb, so you need to be aware when making a choice. Some of the processed and packaged foods include:

- Fast foods

- Margarines

- Ice creams

- Dried foods

- Wheat gluten

- Candies

- Sift drinks and sodas

Artificial sweeteners: This category may seem to be fine as they don't have sugar but people tend to react to them differently, and they also have the potential of affecting the process of ketosis. There are also those who experience a rise in the levels of blood sugar after consuming the artificial sweeteners. Of course, there are options, like Stevia, that are great on a keto diet.

The factory farmed animal protein: It's important that you choose animal protein from grass fed and organic animals. Try to avoid animal protein from the following sources:

- Avoid meat from grain fed animals as they have lower levels of nutrients.

- Avoid the factory farmed fish and pork products as they tend to have high levels of omega six fatty acids which can be inflammatory if consumed in large quantities. The factory farmed fish also tend to have high amounts of mercury which is not suitable for health.

- Avoid consumption of processed meats such as the packaged sausages, hotdogs and such as they contain nitrates which are harmful to the body and can be cancerous.

- Low-fat dairy and milk: Avoid intake of pasteurized milk and the dairy products with reduced fat as they may have high levels of carb content and even contain harmful hormones that are not suitable for the body. Below are some of them to look out for:

- Shredded cheese mostly contain potato starch

- Low fat in dairy products, like the fat-free butter, cream cheese, evaporated skim milk, whipped topping, and the low-fat yogurts. Most of the low fat contains tones of added sugar.

Grains: All grains should be avoided as they have very high amounts of carbohydrates which end up interfering with the process of ketosis.

Fruits: Most fruits should be avoided as they have high levels of sugar and carbs. If you must have fruits, then consider the ones with lower sugar levels like the blackberries and the blueberries.

Starchy vegetables: It's advisable that you avoid all the vegetables that are grown below the ground. These kinds of vegetables have high levels starch which translates to high carbs.

Alcohol: Intake of alcohol can be quite detrimental to the ketogenic process and should be avoided regardless of how difficult it might seem. Many alcoholic drinks have high levels of carbohydrates which are important to note.

Sugars: If you are to succeed in maintaining the process of ketosis then it's advisable that you avoid intake of sugar. So whether it's sugar that's been packaged in products or natural sugar, it still creates the same result and is worth avoiding if you are to stay in ketosis.

Chapter 4
Ketogenic 7 Day Meal Plan

Before you get started with the ketogenic diet, you need a meal plan that you can use as a guide given you may not know which foods to eat when starting out. To be successful with the ketogenic diet, remember, the amount of food that you eat is important. The reason for having a meal plan is to help you ensure that you get in healthy and balanced meals with adequate protein intake, satiation, and fiber.

One of the great things about the ketogenic diet is the fact that it spares loss of muscles as you can burn fat without having to lose muscle mass, leaving you with an appealing physique, especially after weight loss. Keeping to a meal plan allows you to enter ketosis quicker and healthily. Before you get to the meal plan, you have to take time and understand a few guidelines that can help you realize success in the process:

The Ketogenic Meal Plan Guidelines

1. Have a clear guideline on the amount of protein that you need.

Eating the right amount of protein is essential if you are to realize success with the ketogenic diet. Remember, intake of high protein can affect your ketosis process so have a clear understanding of the amount of protein that you should take before planning your meals. It's been recommended that you can have between 10 -25% of protein in your diet, use this range to determine how much protein you should be consuming. Protein is known to help with building and maintaining your muscles, alongside other benefits. To determine the correct amount of protein that you should consume, consider your age, your weight, and how active you are.

If your calorie intake per day is 1500, you can work out the total amount of protein you should consume in a day as follows: 1500x 0.25 = 375. The number of calories that you should consume from protein is 375, and a gram of protein has 4 calories. You would then calculate the grams by dividing, 375/4 = 94. You should, therefore, consume 94 grams of protein per day.

2.   Set the amount of carbs that you need per day

While on the ketogenic diet, it's recommended that your carbohydrate intake is kept at around 5% of your total calories. For example, if your calorie intake per day is 1500 then the exact amount of carbohydrates that you need to take per day is as follows: 1500x .05=75. You are therefore required to consume 75 calories per day. Remember 1 gram of carbohydrates is equivalent to 4 calories. So this is how you can work it out; 75/4=18.75. Your carbohydrate intake will, therefore, be 18.75 grams per day.

7 Day Ketogenic Diet Meal Plan

Day One

Breakfast

- Sausage and Spinach Frittata

- Nutritional Value: Calories 206, Fat 16g, Carbohydrates1 g, protein 12g

- Coffee with heavy cream 2 tablespoons: Calories 120, Fat 12 g, Carbs 1g

Lunch

- Egg salad ½ cup (calories166, fat 14, carbs 1g, protein 10g)

- 4 lettuce leaves (calories 4)

- Cooked bacon 2 slices (calories 92, fat 7g, protein 6g)

Dinner

- Rotisserie chicken 6 oz (calories 276, fat 11g, protein 42)

- Cauliflower gratin ¾ cup (calories 215, fat 19g, net carbs 2g, protein 6g)

- Chopped romaine lettuce 2 cups (calories 16, carbs 1g, protein 1g

- Sugar free salad dressing 2 tablespoons (calories 170, fat 18, carbs 2g, protein 1g)

Day Two

Breakfast

- Spinach frittata and sausage (calories 206, fat 16g,net carbs 2.5g, protein 7g)

Lunch

- Chopped romaine lettuce (calories 16, net carbs 1g, protein 1g)

- Sugar free salad dressing (calories 170, fat 18g, net carbs 2g, protein 1g)

- Chopped leftover chicken (calories 276, fat 11g, protein 42g)

Dinner

- Italian sausage (calories 230, fat 18g, net carbs 1g, protein 13g)

- Cooked broccoli 1 cup (calories 55, net carbs 6, protein 4g)

- Grated parmesan cheese 2 tablespoon (calories 42, fat 3g, protein 4g)

Day Three

Breakfast

- Cream cheese pancakes 2 (calories 172, fat 14g, net carbs 1g, protein 8g)

- Cooked bacon 2 (calories 92, fat 7g, protein 6g)

- Coffee with heavy cream 2 tablespoons (calories 120, fat 12g, net carbs 1g,)

Lunch

- Italian sausage 1 (calories 230, fat 18g, net carbs 1, protein 13g)

- Cauliflower gratin (calories 215, fat 19g, net carbs 2g, protein 6g)

Dinner

- Chili spaghetti casserole (calories 284, fat 20g, net carbs 6g, protein 23g)

- Raw baby spinach 2 cups (calories 14, net carbs 1g, protein 2g)

- Sugar free ranch dressing (calories 70, fat 7g, net carbs 1g)

Day Four

Breakfast

- Sausage and spinach frittata (calories 206, fat 16g, net carbs 1g, protein 12g)

- Coffee with heavy cream 2 tablespoons (calories 206, fat 16g, net carbs 1g, protein 12g)

Lunch

- Spaghetti squash casserole (calories 284, fat 20g, net carbs 6g, protein 23g)

Dinner

- Anti-pasta salad ½ cup (calories 102, fat 8g, net carbs 4g, protein 3g)

- Feta meatballs and sundried tomatoes (calories 356, fat 32g, net carbs 2.5g, protein 24g)

- Baby spinach 2 cups (calories 14, net carbs 1g, protein 2g)

Day Five

Breakfast

- Cream cheese pancakes 2 (calories 172, fat 14g, net carbs 1g, protein 8g)

- Cooked bacon 2pcs (calories 92, fat 7g, protein 6g)

- Coffee with heavy cream (120 calories, fat 12g, net carbs 1g)

Lunch

- Anti pasta salad ½ cup (calories 102, fat 8g, net carbs, 4g, protein 3g)

- Feta meatballs and sundried tomato 4 (calories 356, fat 32g, net carbs 2.5g, protein 24g)

Dinner

- Cuban pot roast 1 cup (calories 271, fat 19g, net carbs 2g, protein 20g)

- Chopped romaine lettuce (calories 16, net carbs 1g, protein 1g)

- Sour cream (calories 51, net carbs 1g, protein 1g)

- Chopped cilantro 1 tablespoon (optional)

- Shredded cheddar cheese ¼ cup (calories 114, fat 4g, net carbs 0.5g, protein 7g)

Day Six

Breakfast

- Scrambled or fried eggs 3 (calories 215, fat 14g, net carbs 1g, protein 19g)

- Butter 1 tablespoon (calories 36)

- Cooked bacon 2 pcs (calories 92, fat 7g, net carbs 1g)

- Coffee with heavy cream (120 calories, fat 12g, net carbs 1g)

Lunch

- Cuban pot roast 1 cup (calories 271, fat 19g, net carbs 2g, protein 20g)

- Chopped romaine lettuce (calories 16, net carbs 1g, protein 1g)

- Sour cream (calories 51, net carbs 1g, protein 1g)

- Chopped cilantro 1 tablespoon (optional)

- Shredded cheddar cheese ¼ cup (calories 114, fat 4g, net carbs 0.5g, protein 7g)

Dinner

- Spaghetti squash casserole (calories 284, fat 20g, net carbs 6g, protein 23g)

- Baby spinach 2 cups (calories 14, net carbs 1g, protein 2g)

- Sugar free ranch dressing (calories 70, fat 7g, net carbs 1g)

Day Seven

Breakfast

- Cream cheese pancakes 2 (calories 172, fat 14g, net carbs 1g, protein 8g)

- Cooked bacon 2pcs (calories 92, fat 7g, protein 6g)

- Coffee with heavy cream (120 calories, fat 12g, net carbs 1g)

Lunch

- Anti pasta salad ½ cup (calories 102, fat 8g, net carbs, 4g, protein 3g)

- Feta meatballs and sundried tomato 4 (calories 356, fat 32g, net carbs 2.5g, protein 24g)

Dinner

- Cuban pot roast 1 cup (calories 271, fat 19g, net carbs 2g, protein 20g)

- Chopped romaine lettuce (calories 16, net carbs 1g, protein 1g)

- Sour cream (calories 51, net carbs 1g, protein 1g)

- Chopped cilantro 1 tablespoon (optional)

- Shredded cheddar cheese ¼ cup (calories 114, fat 4g, net carbs 0.5g, protein 7g)

Chapter 5

Ketogenic Breakfast Recipes

Start off your day with a low carb meal that is both satisfying and nutritious. Eating healthy and nutritious meals gives you the desired energy that you require to stay energized throughout the day. Below are some breakfast recipes that you should try out.

1.   Scrambled Eggs

You can take scrambled eggs with other low carb favorites like sausage, bacon, avocado or your preferred food.

Nutritional Value: Fat 88%, protein 11%, carbs 1%

Cooking time – 5 mins

Serves - 1

Ingredients

- Eggs – 3

- Butter – 2oz

- Salt and Pepper

Instructions

1. Get the eggs whisked together using a fork then add salt and pepper.

2. In a nonstick skillet pour the whisked eggs then stir for about 2 minutes until they appear creamy and cooked.

3. Remove once cooked then serve and enjoy.

2. Frittata with fresh spinach

This low carb recipe is quite a delicacy as you can combine eggs, spinach, sausage, bacon, and vegetables into an amazing breakfast. You can try out the recipe with different types of vegetables.

Nutritional Value: Fat 79%%, protein 19%, carbs 2%

Preparation time – 5 mins Cooking time – 35 mins

Serves – 2

Ingredients

- Eggs – 8

- Heavy whipping cream – 1 cup

- Fresh spinach – ½ lb

- Diced bacon – 1/3 lb

- Butter – 2 tablespoons

- Salt and pepper

Instructions

1. Get the oven preheated to 350F

2. Have the bacon fried with butter until it turns crispy then add the vegetables.

3. Get the eggs whisked together with cream then pour into a baking dish that's greased.

4. Add together spinach, cheese, and bacon on top of the baking dish and then place in the oven as you allow baking for about 30 minutes.

5. Serve and enjoy.

3. Cereal with Cacao Nibs

If you enjoy eating cereal in the morning then this low carb version could be ideal for you. As you switch from your normal diet to a ketogenic diet, you are likely to experience a slight change in your bowel activity and a gut flora imbalance. This keto cereal, with cacao, is ideal as it helps in boosting the level of fiber in your body enhancing bowel activity.

Nutritional Value: Calories 254, Fat 15.5g, protein 9.2g, carbs 1.5g

Preparation time – 10 mins cooking time – 1 hour

Servings - 4

Ingredients

- Chia seeds – ½ cup

- Water – 1 cup

- Hemp hearts – 4 tablespoons

- Fine psyllium powder – 1 tablespoon

- Melted coconut oil – 2 tablespoon

- Organic vanilla extract – 1 tablespoon

- Swerve – 1 tablespoon

- Raw Cacao Nibs – 2 tablespoons.

Instructions

1. Get the oven pre-heated to 285 degrees

2. In a large bowl combine chia seeds with water then get it stirred for about 5 minutes.

3. Add all the ingredients together into the bowl apart from the

cacao nibs. You can then breakdown the nibs into smaller pieces then add them too.

4. Mix all the ingredients together using an electric mixer or even a wooden spoon until well combined.

5. F you prefer the cacao nibs in bigger chunks then you can have them mixed at this stage then stir accordingly. The mixture should then form a nice consistent ball.

6. Roll out two oven papers that are large enough then form the dough into cylindrical shapes using your hands. Place the formed cylindrical dough on the parchment paper with the shiny side facing upwards.

7. Use your fingers to flatten the dough then cover it with the other paper then use a rolling pin to roll out to a thickness of about 18 inches.

8. Peel off the top paper gently then on a cookie sheet lay the dough then allow to bake until almost dry or for about 15 minutes.

9. Once ready remove from oven as you also take off the sheet from the dough.

10. Bake it again for about 15 more minutes then remove and allow to cool.

11. Use a large knife to cut the cereals into smaller square pieces then serve and enjoy or get it stored in an airtight container for a period of 3 days.

4. Grain free hemp heart porridge

This is a delicious meal that is gluten free and sugar-free making it perfect for those on a ketogenic diet.

Nutritional Value: Calories 867, Fat 72.8g, protein 43.8g, Net carbs 2.3g, Sugar 5g

Preparation time – 10 mins cooking time – 1 hour

Servings - 3

Ingredients

- Non-dairy milk – 1 cup

- Manitoba harvest hemp hearts – ½ cup

- Flax seed freshly ground – 2 tablespoons

- Chia seeds – 1 tablespoon

- Alcohol-free stevia – 1 tablespoon

- Pure vanilla extract

- Ground Cinnamon – ½ teaspoon

- Almond flour – ¼ cup

Toppings

- Brazil nuts – 3

- Manitoba harvest hemp hearts – 1 tablespoon

Instructions

1. In a saucepan, add all the ingredients apart from the toppings and the almonds. Stir in the mixture until well mixed.

2. Place the mixture over medium heat and allow it to heat to a

boil.

3. Remove from heat then add in the crushed almonds. Serve in a bowl and add the toppings.

4. Enjoy immediately.

5. Almond Joy Pancakes

Nutritional Value: Fat 17g, protein 11g, Net carbs 17g

Preparation time – 10 mins Cooking time – 10 mins

Servings – 6

Ingredients

- Coconut flour – 1/.2 cup

- Unsweetened shredded coconut – 1/3 cup

- Sweetener of choice – ¼ cup

- Baking powder – 1/2teaspoon

- Salt – ½ tablespoon

- Large eggs – 6

- Melted coconut oil – ¼ cup

- Unsweetened almond milk – ½ cup

- Almond extract – 1 tablespoon

- Toasted slivered almonds – ¼ cup

- Finely Chopped Cacao Chocolate – 2 ounces

Instructions

1. Mix together in a large bowl of coconut flour, baking powder, sweetener and shredded coconut and salt.

2. Stir the eggs in coconut oil, almond milk ½ cup, and almond extract. Add almond milk as required. The batter mixture

should be thicker when compared to the traditional pancake batter.

3. Add in the chopped chocolate and toasted almonds.

4. Over medium heat place a large skillet then brush it through with coconut oil or your preferred cooking oil. Add two scoops of butter to the skillet then spread to form a circle of about 4 inches.

5. Cook the pancakes until golden brown on the bottom with the top edges well set.

6. Continue with the cooking until the other side also gets golden brown.

7. Remove from the pan when ready and allow to stay warm. You can repeat the same process with the remaining batter.

8. Serve and enjoy

6. Bacon and Avocado

Nutritional Value: Calories 313, Fat 26 g, protein 11, Net carbs 17g

Preparation time – 2 mins Cooking time – 12 mins

Servings – 2

Ingredients

- Uncured pastured bacon - 4 strips

- Large avocado, peeled and cut into slices – 1

- Large Organic Eggs – 2

- Sea salt – ¼

Instructions

1. Place the avocado and bacon into a frying pan over medium heat.

2. Allow the avocado and bacon to fry as you flip after each 3 minutes.

3. Remove the bacon and avocado then set aside once cooked.

4. leave the bacon fat in the pan and crack your eggs in.

5. Fry the eggs for about 3 minutes then flip and allow to fry until the right consistency is attained.

6. Serve and enjoy.

7. Green Buttered Eggs

Nutritional Value: Calories 311, Fat 27.5 g, protein 12.8g, Net carbs 2.5 g Fiber 1 g

Preparation time – 5 mins Cooking time – 12 mins

Servings – 2

Ingredients

- Pastured organic butter – 2 tablespoons

- Coconut oil - 1 tablespoon

- Finely chopped garlic cloves – 2

- Fresh thyme leaves – 1 tablespoon

- Chopped fresh cilantro – ½ cup

- Organic eggs – 4

- Ground cumin

- Ground Cayenne

- Sea salt – ½ teaspoon

Instructions

1. Use a non-stick skillet to melt coconut oil and butter as you allow it to heat for a minute.

2. Add into the skillet chopped garlic then cook for 3 minutes. Add thyme and cook for 30 seconds until it browns. Remember not to burn the garlic.

3. Add parsley and cilantro then cook for 3 minutes until it becomes crisp. Crack the eggs right into the pan as you ensure that the yoke remains unbroken.

4. Get the pan covered with a lid as you lower the heat to low. Let it cook for 6 minutes until the yolk is well set.

5. Serve once cooked and enjoy

8. Cheddar and Chive Soufflés

Nutritional Value: Calories 212, Fat 23.6 g, protein 14g, Net carbs 2.3g, Fiber 1g

Preparation time – 10 mins Cooking time – 35 mins

Servings – 8 soufflés

Ingredients

- Almond flour – 1/ cup

- Salt – 1 teaspoon

- Ground Mustard – 1 teaspoon

- Black Pepper – ½ teaspoon

- Xanthan gum – 1/ teaspoon

- Cayenne pepper – ¼ teaspoon

- Heavy Cream - ¾ cup

- Shredded cheddar cheese – 2 cups

- Chopped fresh Chives – ¼ cup

- Large eggs – 6

- Cream of tartar – ¼ teaspoon

- Dash salt

Instructions

1. Get the oven pre-heated to 350F then grease the ramekins and set on a cookie sheet.

2. Whisk together almond flour, pepper, mustard, salt, cayenne

and xantham gum in a large bowl. Slowly add the cream until all is well combined.

3. Add cheese, egg yolks, and chives into the mixture, mix well.

4. In a separate bowl, mix the egg whites with cream of tartar then add salt and stir until the mixture becomes glossy.

5. Fold the egg whites into the almond flour and cheese mixture until well combined.

6. Divide the mixture into the prepared ramekins then place the cookie sheets carefully into the preheated oven.

7. Allow the mixture to bake for 25 minutes or until the soufflés rises to an inch above the rim and are browned.

8. Serve and enjoy

9. Swiss Chard and Ricotta Pie

Nutritional Value: Calories 344, Fat 27 g, protein 23g, Net carbs 4g.

Preparation time – 8 mins Cooking time – 35 mins

Servings - 2

Ingredients

- Olive oil – 1 tablespoon
- Chopped onion – 1 cup
- Minced clove garlic – 1
- Chopped swiss chard - 8 cups
- Ricotta cheese – 2 cups
- Eggs – 3
- Shredded Mozzarella – 1 cup
- Shredded Parmesan – ¼ cup
- Ground Nutmeg – 1/8 teaspoon
- Salt and pepper
- Mild Sausage – 1 lb

Instructions

1. In a large pan heat oil then add garlic and onions. Allow to cook for a few minutes then add swiss chard or your preferred greens.

2. Cook for 5 minutes until the leaves get wilted and the stems soft. Add in nutmeg then season with pepper and salt. Remove from the heat then set aside.

3. In a separate bowl whisk the eggs then add ricotta, mozzarella cheese, and parmesan. Add in the sautéed greens then stir.

4. In case you are making a large pie then you can roll out the sausage then press it uniformly into the pie tin.

5. Pour the filling then place it on a cooking sheet. Allow it to bake at 350F for 30 minutes or until it gets firm.

10.   Egg Fat Breakfast Biscuit

Nutritional Value: Calories 572, Fat 53 g, protein 21g, Net carbs 3g, Fiber 2g

Preparation time – 8 mins Cooking time – 35 mins

Servings - 2

Ingredients

- Softened cream cheese – 1 ounce

- Grated parmesan cheese – 2tablespoons

- Baking powder – 1/8 teaspoon

- Unfiltered apple cider vinegar – ½ teaspoon

- Kosher salt – 1 pinch

- Black pepper freshly ground

- Large eggs – 2 separate 1

- Extra virgin olive oil – 2 tablespoon

- Deli deluxe American Cheese – ½ slice

Instructions

1. Soften the cream cheese then blend with baking powder, parmesan, apple cider vinegar, granulated garlic, kosher salt and egg whites for one egg.

2. Add olive oil ½ teaspoon to two ramekins then divide the batter and nuke for about 35 seconds while in the microwave. The centers should not be put in the middle

3. Into a non-stick skillet, add ½ teaspoon of olive oil the transfer egg biscuits the allow to cook until well toasted.

4. Remove from the pan then top each half with a slice of American cheese. Allow it to melt as you fry the egg.

5. In a non-stick skillet, add the remaining oil then add the remaining egg with egg yolk from the other egg. Allow it to fry until the whites are firm and yolk runny.

6. Add the egg to the bottom of the biscuit then top with another biscuit.

7. Serve and enjoy.

11. Avocado and Salmon

Nutritional Value: Calories 525, Fat 48 g, protein 19g, Net carbs 4g.

Preparation time – 5 mins Cooking time –5 mins

Servings - 1

Ingredients

- Ripe organic avocado – 1 ripe

- Smoked salmon wild caught – 60grams

- Fresh and soft goat cheese – 30 grams

- Extra virgin olive oil – 2 tablespoons

- Lemon Juice – 1 lemon

- Sea salt – a pinch

Instructions

1. Have the avocado cut into two and the seed removed.

2. Mix all the remaining ingredients together in a food processor until they get coarsely chopped.

3. Place the cream into the avocado then cut the avocado into smaller cubes. Cut the salmon also into small pieces then have the two mixed together.

4. Add goat cheese, and the remaining ingredients then blend well.

12. Keto White Pizza Frittata

Nutritional Value: Calories 298, Fat 23.8g, protein 19.4 g, Net carbs 2.1 g.

Preparation time – 10 mins Cooking time –25 mins

Servings – 8 Slices

Ingredients

- Large eggs – 12

- Frozen Spinach – 9 0z

- Pepperoni – 1 oz

- Minced Garlic – 5 oz

- Minced Garlic – 1 teaspoon

- Fresh Ricotta Cheese – ½ cup

- Parmesan Cheese – ½ cup

- Olive Oil – 1/ tablespoon

- Nutmeg – ¼ tablespoon

- Salt and pepper

Instructions

1. Microwave spinach that's frozen for 4 minutes or until defrosted. Drain as much water as you can from the spinach by squeezing with your hands then set aside.

2. Pre-heat the oven to about 375F

3. Mix all the eggs together with spices, and olive oil then whisk until well combined.

4. Add ricotta cheese, spinach, and parmesan cheese then break the spinach into small pieces as you add.

5. Pour the mixture into a skillet then sprinkle mozzarella cheese on top and pepperoni.

6. Bake for about 30 minutes or until completely set.

7. You can top it up with your favorite fatty sauce then serve and joy.

Chapter 6

Ketogenic Lunch Recipes

1.   Chicken Pad Thai

Nutritional Value: Calories 710, Fat 34g, protein 90 g, Net carbs 13g.

Preparation time – 20 mins Cooking time –10 mins

Servings – 4

Ingredients

- Ground ginger – 1/8 teaspoon

- Garlic powder – 1/8 teaspoon

- Black pepper freshly ground – 1/8 teaspoon

- Free range chicken – 2 pounds

- Peanut oil – 2 tablespoons

- Free range eggs – 3 large

- Organic chicken broth – 1/3 cup

- Peanut butter - 3 tablespoons

- Tamari – 2 tablespoons

- Rice Vinegar – 1 tablespoon

- Chopped scallion – ½ cup

- Minced garlic cloves – 2

- Red pepper flakes – 1 teaspoon

- Spiralized zucchini – 4

- Bean sprouts – 1/ cup

- Crushed peanuts for garnish - ½ cup

- Lime for garnish cut into wedges - 1

Instructions

1. Mix together in a medium bowl garlic powder, ginger, salt and black pepper. Add chicken tenders then toss until well coated.

2. Heat in a medium skillet peanut oil then add chicken tenders once the oil becomes hot. Allow to cook for 3 minutes as you turn once.

3. Remove chicken from skillet once cooked then cut into thick slices of about ¼ inch.

4. Add eggs into the skillet then scramble for about 1 minute. Remove from the skillet once ready then set aside.

5. Reduce the heat to low then add chicken broth, tamari, vinegar, chicken broth, pepper flakes and peanut butter then stir well and allow to cook for about 3 minutes.

6. Add the slices of chicken, zucchini noodles, sprouts and scrambled eggs then toss to coat with well with the sauce and allow to cook for about 1 minute.

7. Serve the pad thai then garnish with lime wedges and peanuts.

2. Crockpot Chicken Stew

Nutritional Value: Calories 228, Fat 11g, protein 23g, Net carbs 6g.

Preparation time – 5 mins Cooking time – 2 hours

Servings – 4

Ingredients

- Chicken stock – 2 cups

- Medium Carrots diced and finely peeled – ½ cup

- Skinless and boneless chicken thighs diced – 28 ounces

- Spring fresh rosemary - 1

- Minced garlic cloves – 3

- Dried thyme – ¼ teaspoon

- Dried oregano – ½ teaspoon

- Fresh spinach – 1 cup

- Heavy cream – ½ cup

- Salt and pepper

- Xanthum gum – 1/8 teaspoon

Instructions

1. Place chicken stock, celery, carrots, onions, chicken thighs, garlic, thyme, and rosemary into a larger Crockpot then allow to cook for about 2 hours over high heat.

2. Add pepper and salt to taste then stir in the heavy cream and spinach.

3. Sprinkle the chicken with xantham gum to the desired thickness.

4. Whisk, mix and cook for an extra 10 minutes then serve and enjoy.

3. Vegan Sesame Tofu and Eggplant

Nutritional Value: Calories 292, Fat 25g, protein 11 g, Net carbs 6g.

Preparation time – 20 mins cooking time –10 mins

Servings – 4

Ingredients

- Block firm tofu – 1 pound

- Chopped cilantro – 1 cup

- Rice vinegar – 3 tablespoons

- Toasted sesame oil – 4 tablespoons

- Finely minced cloves garlic – 2

- Crushed red pepper flakes – 1 teaspoon

- Swerve confectioners – 2 teaspoons

- Eggplant – 1 whole

- Salt and pepper

- Sesame seeds – ¼ cup

- Soy sauce – ¼ cup

Instructions

1. Get the oven pre-heated to 200F

2. Remove the tofu then get it wrapped in paper towels then press some weight on it so as to press water out.

3. In a large mixing bowl, place cilantro, rice vinegar toasted sesame oil, crushed red pepper, minced garlic and red pepper

flakes then whisk all together.

4. Peel the egg plant then julienne and then mix the eggplant with marinade.

5. Place a skillet over medium heat then add olive oil and cook the egg plants for about 3 minutes or until it becomes soft.

6. Add cilantro to the eggplant then transfer to a safe dish in the oven. Cover the dish then place in the oven to keep warm then wipe the skillet and place it on the heat again.

7. Unwrap and cut the tofu into 8 slices then have the sesame seeds spread on a plate. Press the tofu onto the seeds on both sides.

8. Add sesame oil into the skillet then fry tofu for 5 minutes on both sides or until the tofu turns crisp. Add soy sauce to the pan then coat tofu in it. Allow it to cook until the tofu gets browned.

9. Remove the noodles then serve on a plate. Place tofu on top of the noodles then enjoy.

4. Salmon Patties with Fresh herbs

Nutritional Value: Calories 418, Fat 25g, protein 46 g, Net carbs 2.6g.

Preparation time – 10 mins cooking time –15 mins

Servings – 5

Ingredients

- Pink salmon – 2 cans

- Chopped fresh chives – 2 tablespoons

- Chopped fresh dill – ¼ cup

- Grated parmesan cheese – ¼ cup

- Crushed pork rinds – 4 ounces

- Large eggs – 2

- Lemon zest – 1 teaspoon

- Salt pepper

- Almond pepper – ½ cup

- Olive oil – 2 tablespoons

Instructions

1. Unpack salmon then add to a large mixing bowl.

2. Mix the chives, parmesan cheese, dill, crushed pork rinds, lemon zest, salt, pepper, and eggs into salmon then mix together.

3. Form salmon into balls of about 3 ounces, you are more likely to get 10 balls.

4. Place almond flour into a plate then in your hands flatten the salmon patty then dip into the flour.

5. Over medium heat place the skillet then add olive oil and allow to heat for a few minutes. Place the salmon patty and cook until browned.

6. You can then serve the salmon with veggies or homemade tartar sauce.

5.   Lamb Meatballs with Cauliflower Pilaf

Nutritional Value: Calories 495, Fat 41g, protein 27 g, Net carbs 3.5g.

Preparation time – 5 mins cooking time –30 mins

Servings – 4

Ingredients

- Cauliflower florets – 200 grams

- Salt and pepper

- Ground lamb – 1 lb

- Large egg – 1

- Fennel seed – 1 teaspoon

- Garlic powder – 1 teaspoon

- Paprika – 1 teaspoon

- Coconut oil – 2 tablespoon

- Chopped yellow onion – ½

- Minced garlic – 4 grams

- Fresh mint leaves – 1 bunch

- Lemon zest – 1 tablespoon

- Goat Cheese – 4 oz

Instructions

1. Pulse the cauliflower into a food processor until it gets to look like rice then cook in an oiled pan for about 8 minutes as you also season with salt and pepper to taste.

2. Combine in a large bowl egg, lamb and spices then mix well using your hands then form about 12 meatballs. Set aside the meat balls.

3. Place a skillet over medium heat then add onion and coconut oil. Allow to cook for about 8 minutes or until it gets translucent.

4. Add the meatballs to the cooking pan then cook the meatballs on all sides until they become firm with no pink look.

5. Divide the cauliflower into 4 portions then add some meatballs to each of the cauliflower portions.

6. Top it up with lemon zest, fresh mint leaves, and the crumbled goat cheese.

7. Enjoy.

6. Cheesy Spinach Rolls with Apple Slaw

Nutritional Value: Calories 670, Fat 67, protein 32g, Net carbs 16g.

Preparation time – 35 mins cooking time – 15 mins

Servings – 16 rolls

Ingredients

Crust

- Shredded mozzarella - 2.5 cups
- Almond Flour – ½ cup
- Coconut flour – 6 tablespoon
- Large Eggs – 2
- Sea salt

Filling

- Spinach – 6 oz
- Cream cheese - 4oz
- Grated parmesan – ¼ pinch
- Sea salt – 1 pinch

Topping

- Cole slaw salad mix – ¾
- Apple – 1
- Mayonnaise – ¼ cup
- Sea salt – ¼ teaspoon

Instructions

1. Get the oven preheated to 350F

2. Place a large pan over medium heat then add olive or avocado oil, spinach leaves then allow to cook until wilted.

3. Add parmesan, cream cheese and then stir until well melted and combined.

4. Take it off the heat and put it aside as you prepare the crust.

5. For the crust; microwave mozzarella cheese for about 30 seconds or until it gets soft.

6. Add coconut oil and almond flour then mix. Add eggs, salt and then mix well. It takes a few minutes for it to mix well.

7. Once the mixture gains consistency lay it on a sheet of parchment on the countertop. Place another parchment paper on top of the dough then flatten it using a rolling pin to about 1/8 inches thickness.

8. Use a sharp knife or a pizza cutter to cut the dough into rectangles of 3" x 4" or as desired. Add the ½ teaspoon of the prepared spinach mixture to one side f the rectangle then fold the dough carefully as you roll it into a cigar shape.

9. Transfer the rolls to a baking sheet that's lined with greased parchment paper.

10. Pin the ends of the rolls to create a seal then bake the rolls for about 18 minutes or until they turn golden brown.

11. Allow them to cool once ready for about 10 minutes

12. To make apple slaw, grate 1 apple then place in a mixing bowl. Add cole slaw salad then mix together with salt and mayonnaise.

13. Mix all well then refrigerate until ready.

14. Serve the rolls as you top them with apple slaw mix then enjoy.

7. Low Carb Chicken Quesadilla

Nutritional Value: Calories 654, Fat 43, protein 52g, Net carbs 7g.

Preparation time – 5 mins cooking time – 5mins

Servings – 1

Ingredients

- Pepper jack – 3 oz

- Grilled chicken breast – 2.5 oz

- Sliced thin avocado – ½

- Chopped jalapeno – 1 teaspoon

- Low carb wrap – 1

Spices

- Dried basil – ¼ teaspoon

- Crushed red pepper – ¼ teaspoon

- Garlic powder – ¼ teaspoon

- Salt – ¼ teaspoon

Instructions

1. Grill the chicken breasts alongside spices for added flavor. Ensure that the chicken breasts are chopped for faster cooking.

2. On a wide frying pan, place the wrap and allow it to lay fully flat over medium heat.

3. Add chopped chicken breast, jalapeno, sliced avocado to half of the wrap.

4. Use a spatula to fold the other wrap as you press it down to flatten. The pressing ensures that the melted cheese sticks with the quesadilla well.

5. Take it off the pan and then cut into thirds. You can go ahead and enjoy with some sour cream or salsa.

8. Chipotle Steak bowl

Nutritional Value: Calories 620, Fat 50, protein 33g, Net carbs 5.5g.

Preparation time – 15 mins cooking time – 8mins

Servings – 4

Ingredients

- Skirt steak – 16 oz

- Salt and pepper

Guacamole

- Avocados – 2

- Diced red onion- ¼ cup

- Grape tomatoes – 6

- Clove garlic – 1

- Olive oil – 1 tablespoon

- Fresh cilantro

- Lime – 1

- Crushed red pepper – 1/8 tablespoon

- Pepper jack cheese – 4 oz

- Sour cream – 1 cup

- Fresh cilantro – 1 handful

- Chipotle Tabasco sauce – 1 splash

Instructions

1. Get the skirt steak seasoned with salt and pepper then place it in a skillet over high heat. Allow the steak to cook for about 4 minutes on both sides then let it rest as you prepare guacamole.

2. To prepare the guacamole: Cut the avocados then mash in a mixing bowl.

3. Dice the tomatoes and red onions then add to your avocado.

4. Squeeze garlic clove then mix to combine with olive oil

5. Add cilantro and lime juice then season with salt, pepper, and crushed red pepper to taste. Mix well then set aside.

6. Slice the steak with the grain into small sized strips then divide into about 4 potions.

7. Have the pepper jack cheese shredded then use it to top each of the skirt steak.

8. Splash each portion with fresh cilantro and chipotle Tabasco sauce.

9. Serve with guacamole and enjoy.

9. Low Carb Garlic Shrimp Pasta

Nutritional Value: Calories 360, Fat 21, protein 36g, Net carbs 3.5g.

Preparation time – 10 mins cooking time – 10 mins

Servings – 4

Ingredients

- Miracle Noodle – 2 bags

- Butter – 2 tablespoon

- Olive oil – 2 tablespoon

- Cloves garlic – 4

- Lemon – ½

- Large raw shrimp – 1 lb

- Paprika – ½ teaspoon

- Fresh basil

- Salt and pepper

Instructions

1. Place the noodles into a pot of water then remove and rinse. Place the noodles in cool water and allow to stay for about 2 minutes.

2. Place a cooking pan over medium heat then add the noodles and roast them until all the excess water is removed then set aside once dry.

3. Add olive oil and butter to the same pan then heat. Add crushed garlic cloves then cook until fragrant.

4. Have the lemons sliced into rounds then add the shrimp and lemon slices to the cooked garlic. Allow to cook for 3 minutes as you turn the shrimps on all sides.

5. Once the shrimps are cooked, add noodles to the pan then season with paprika, pepper, and salt.

6. Toss everything to coat the noodles well then serves.

7. Sprinkle basil on top then enjoy

10.   Green Bean Fries

Nutritional Value: Calories 113, Fat 6, protein 9g, Net carbs 2.5g.

Preparation time – 10 mins cooking time – 10 mins

Servings – 4

Ingredients

- Green beans – 12 oz

- Large egg – 1

- Grated Parmesan – 2/3 cup

- Himalayan salt – ½ cup

- Black Pepper – ¼ teaspoon

- Garlic powder – ½ teaspoon

- Paprika – ¼ teaspoon

Instructions

1. Get the oven preheated to 400F

2. Ensure the green beans are snipped and dry then on a shallow plate mix grated parmesan cheese with all the seasonings until evenly mixed.

3. Whisk an egg in the bowl and have the green beans drenched in it. Once the beans are drenched, allow the excess to drop off then gently press the beans into the cheese mixture as you also sprinkle some cheese over.

4. Toss with your hands gently then place on a greased baking sheet as

5. You ensure there is sufficient room for them to crisp on all

sides.

6. Bake for 10 minutes then check to see if the cheese has turned golden.

7. Once the beans are baked, allow them to cool then serve with some spicy ranch or mayo.

11. Easy Buffalo Wings

Nutritional Value: Calories 620, Fat 46, protein 48g, Net carbs 1g.

Preparation time – 1o mins cooking time – 20 mins

Servings – 2

Ingredients

- Chicken wings - 6

- Butter – 2 tablespoon

- Red hot sauce – ½ cup

- Salt and pepper

- Garlic powder - ½ teaspoon

- Paprika – ½ teaspoon

- Cayenne (Optional)

Instructions

1. Break the chicken wing into two pieces then pour red hot sauce over the wings to coat them lightly.

2. Season the wings and toss them then refrigerate for 1 hour as you move to the next step.

3. Turn your broiler to high heat then place the rack at 6 inches above the broiler. Line the baking sheet using aluminum paper then place the chicken wings as you allow sufficient space so that both sides can get enough heat.

4. Let the wings cook for 8 minutes or until the wings begin to turn dark brown.

5. Melt butter and the remaining red hot sauce. You can also add

cayenne pepper and once the butter is melted remove off the heat.

6. Take the wings out of the broiler then flip them into the sauce then return them again to the broiler and allow to cook for about 8 minutes.

7. Once the wings brown on both sides place them in a bowl then pour on them the hot sauce as you toss to evenly coat them.

8. Enjoy them with carrots, celery or bleu cheese.

12. Juicy Butter Burgers

Nutritional Value: Calories 443, Fat 34, protein 25g, Net carbs 4g.

Preparation time – 10 mins cooking time – 8 mins

Servings – 2

Ingredients

- Ground beef – ½ lb

- Strip bacon – 1

- Sliced pickled jalapenos – 1 tablespoon

- Mayo – 1 tablespoon

- Plum tomato – ½

- Onion – ¼

- Sriracha - 1 tablespoon

- Egg – 1

- Butter – 2 tablespoon

- Lettuce leaves – 2

Spices

- Salt – ½ teaspoon

- Crushed red pepper – ½ teaspoon

- Cayenne – ¼ teaspoon

- Basil – ½ teaspoon

Instructions

1. Press, fold and stretch the meat for 3 minutes to make it more sticky when adding the ingredients.

2. Dice and chop all the ingredients then add all the diced ingredients to the meat and knead until you get a uniform consistency.

3. Divide the meatballs into 4 pieces then add butter at the center of two of the meatballs. Seal the sides as you prepare it for grilling.

4. Place the patties in the pan, you can also add onions then allow to cook as you flip after 5 minutes.

5. Flip the onions on both sides. The burger should then be ready. You can then serve them as you lay pieces of lettuce with mayo on them.

6. Use your choice toppings to top them up alongside the caramelized onions, sliced tomato, sriracha, sliced jalapeno and some more mayo.

7. Cheese and ketchup can also be used for a more traditional taste.

8. Enjoy

Chapter 7

Ketogenic Dinner Recipes

1. Lemon Rosemary Chicken with Roasted Broccolini

Nutritional Value: Calories 289, Fat 14, protein 30g, Net carbs 12g, fiber 4g.

Preparation time – 10 mins cooking time – 45 mins

Servings – 4

Ingredients

- Chopped fresh parsley – 2 tablespoons

- Chopped fresh rosemary – 1 ½ tablespoon

- Chopped garlic clove – 1 large

- Dijon Mustard – 2 tablespoon

- Olive oil – 3 tablespoons

- Kosher salt

- Freshly ground black pepper

- Lemon cut into slices – 1

- Chicken breasts - 2 ½ lbs

- Red onion – ½ wedges

- Crushed red pepper – ½ teaspoon

Instructions

1. Get the oven preheated to 4250F

2. In a large bowl combine rosemary, parsley, garlic, dijon then add oil and season with black pepper and salt.

3. Place the slices of lemon and part of rosemary mixture into the chicken then rub the remaining mixture over chicken.

4. Roast the chicken on rimmed baking sheet for about 20 minutes.

5. In a bowl toss red pepper, broccolini onion and lemon slices then add black pepper and oil as you season with salt.

6. Remove the baking sheet then arrange the vegetables around the chicken. Allow to bake for about 15 minutes.

7. Serve the chicken as you sprinkle with red pepper.

2. Crockpot Double Beef

Nutritional Value: Calories 222, Fat 7, protein 27g, Net carbs 9g.

Preparation time – 15 mins cooking time – 35 mins

Servings – 4

Ingredients

- Beef stew meat – 1.5lbs

- Diced tomatoes – 214.5 oz

- Chili mix – 1 tablespoon

- Beef broth – 1 cup

- Worcestershire sauce salt

Instructions

1. Set the crockpot to high then add all the ingredients together and mix.

2. Allow to cook on high for about 45 minutes then add salt to taste and cook again for 10 minutes.

3. Serve and enjoy

3.   Roasted Brussels Sprouts with Bacon

Nutritional Value: Calories 278, Fat 21, protein 15g, Net carbs 4g.

Preparation time – 5 mins cooking time – 30 mins

Servings – 4

Ingredients

- Brussels sprouts – 1 lb

- Olive oil – 2 tablespoons

- Strips bacon – 8 trips

- Salt

- Pepper

Instructions

1. Get the oven preheated to 3750F

2. Cut the ends of the Brussels sprout then cut them in half or quarter if big enough.

3. Place them into a bowl then toss with olive oil, pepper, and salt. You can toss them in cumin and red pepper.

4. On a greased baking sheet place the Brussels sprouts as you ensure there is sufficient space in between them as you roast them nicely.

5. Place the baking sheet in the oven as you allow top bake for about 30 minutes. Once half way through shaking the sheet so that the Brussels sprouts can rotate well.

6. As the brussels sprouts get baked, fry bacon then once ready chop into small pieces.

7. Once the Brussel sprouts are ready, toss them with the cooked bit sized bacon

8. Serve on a large plate then sprinkle with salt and enjoy.

4. Roasted Garlic and Rosemary Cauliflower Mash

Nutritional Value: Calories 200, Fat 16, protein 4g, Net carbs 7g.

Preparation time – 30 mins cooking time – 10 mins

Servings – 4

Ingredients

- Cloves garlic – 4 cloves

- Olive oil – 1 tablespoon

- Cauliflower – ½ 800g

- Butter – 4tablespoon

- Rosemary – 1 tablespoon

- Salt and pepper

Instructions

- Roast the garlic cloves then place in an aluminum tray. Drizzle them with olive oil then bake at 400F for 12 minutes

- Cut cauliflower into small sizes then place over simmering water as you ensure that the lid of the steam basket fits well.

- Steam them for 10 minutes or until you can easily pierce through them easily.

- Drain water from the pot then return the cauliflower back into the pot. Add all the seasonings and the roasted garlic cloves.

- Blend the mixture well until creamy and smooth.

- Serve and enjoy

5. Lemon Garlic Shrimp Kabobs

Nutritional Value: Calories 189, Fat 7, protein 31 g, Net carbs 2g.

Preparation time – 10 mins cooking time – 10 mins

Servings – 6

Ingredients

- Peeled and deveined medium shrimp – 1 ½
- Thinly sliced lemons - 4 (halved)
- Kosher salt
- Black pepper freshly ground
- Unsalted butter – ¼ cup
- Lemon juice freshly squeezed – ¼
- Minced cloves garlic – 4
- Dried oregano – ½ teaspoon
- Dried thyme – ½
- Dried basil – ½ teaspoon
- Chopped fresh parsley – 2 tablespoons

Instructions

1. Get the oven preheated to 450F
2. Coat the baking sheet with non-stick spray then get the lemon and shrimp threaded then placed on the baking sheet.
3. Place then into the oven then roast for about 7 minutes or until firm and well cooked.

4. In a medium skillet melt butter over high heat then stir in garlic, lemon juice, thyme, oregano and basil until fragrant then season with pepper and salt to taste.

5. Serve the shrimp skewers as you brush them with butter mixture. You can also garnish with parsley or as desired.

6. Low Carb Skillet Brownies

Nutritional Value: Calories 333, Fat 31, protein 6g, Net carbs 3g.

Preparation time – 15 mins cooking time – 30 mins

Servings – 4

Ingredients

Brownies

- Butter – 6 tablespoons
- Erythritol – 1/3 cup
- Cocoa Powder - 1/3 cup
- Egg – 1
- Vanilla Extract – ½ teaspoon
- Salt
- Almond Flour – ¼ teaspoon
- Baking Powder ½ teaspoon
- Walnuts – ¼ cup

Drizzle

- Peanut butter – 1 tablespoon
- Butter – 1 tablespoon

Instructions

1. Get the oven preheated to 350F

2. On a small pan melt butter and erythritol or your preferred granulated sweetener then allow it to dissolve in the butter.

3. Pour the combination of butter and erythritol into a bowl then add salt, vanilla extract and cocoa powder. Add in egg then whisk until well combined.

4. Add in almond flour alongside baking powder to make the brownie rise a little bit.

5. You can fold in any add ins or your choice nuts like walnuts for enhanced brownie taste.

6. Pour the brownie batter into cast iron skillet.

7. To prepare the drizzle, melt peanut butter and butter in a small span then pour it on the brownie batter then allow to bake for 30 minutes then remove to cool.

8. Serve and enjoy.

7. Prawn and Chorizo Frittata

Nutritional Value: Calories 387 , Fat 25, protein 34 g, Net carbs 8g.

Preparation time – 10 mins cooking time – 25 mins

Servings – 2

Ingredients

- Finely chopped onions – ½ tablespoon

- Sliced chorizo – 50g

- Olive oil – 2 tablespoon

- Eggs – 4

- Milk – 1 tablespoon

- Cooked peeled prawn – 85g

- Defrosted frozen pea – 100g

- Leafy salad

Instructions

1. Have the grill heated to medium heat then in a frying pan add add onion, chorizo and oil then fry for about 5 minutes as you occasionally stir until the onion becomes soft.

2. Remove the pan out of the heat then drain out excess fat. Stir into the pan whisked eggs, milk and some seasoning.

3. Add prawns and peas then reduce heat to low as you allow to cook for about 10 minutes or until the frittata top is set.

4. Place it under the grill until it gets golden then remove and serve in wedges with some leafy salad.

8. Cheese and Onion pork chops

Nutritional Value: Calories 378, Fat 23, protein 36 g, Net carbs 8g.

Preparation time – 5 mins cooking time – 15 mins

Servings – 4

Ingredients

- Pork chops – 4

- Olive Oil – 2 tablespoons

- English Mustard – 1 tablespoon

- Caramelized Onions – 4 tablespoons

- Grated Cheshire cheese - 50g

- Chopped thyme – 1 tablespoon

Instructions

1. Have the grill heated to high then place the pork chops on a grill pan then rub with oil as you also season. Allow to grill for about 6 minutes as you turn on all sides or until golden.

2. Spread mustard over one side of the chops then top with onions. Have cheese and thyme mixed together the sprinkle the mixture over the pork chops.

3. Let it grill until golden or bubbly.

4. Serve and enjoy

9. Seafood Curry

Nutritional Value: Calories 189, Fat 7, protein 31 g, Net carbs 2g.

Preparation time – 10 mins cooking time – 35 mins

Servings – 6

Ingredients

- Ghee – 75g

- Skinless white fish – 300g

- Skinless salmon – 200g

- Raw peeled prawn – 200g

- Mussels cleaned and debearded – 100g

For Curry Sauce

- Roughly chopped onion – 1

- Chopped ginger – 100g

- Vegetable oil – 50ml

- Garam masala – 2 tablespoon

- Tumeric – 1 teaspoon

- Deseeded Red chili – 1

- Chopped canned tomatoes – 400g

- Coriander leaves – handful

Instructions

1. For curry sauce: Mix ginger and onion together into a puree then in a large pan heat oil then add garam marsala as you

allow to sizzle for about 30 seconds. Add the ginger and onion puree then allow to cook for about 5 minutes over medium heat.

2. Add all the remaining ingredients then fry for about 1 minute add chili and tomatoes then fry for 1 minute. Add salt and pepper then stir well.

3. Melt part of the ghee in a pan then cook the white fish for about 3 minutes or until browned lightly. Set it aside on a plate once cooked.

4. Follow the same process for the prawns and salmon as you add ghee each time you are cooking. As for the mussels place a medium sized pan over high heat then add the mussels and water.

5. Cover the lid tightly and allow to steam for about 4 minutes as you shake the pan in the process.

6. Drain the mussels then set aside with others.

7. Bring the sauce to boiling point then stir in the mussels and fish gently. Allow all to boil for about 4 minutes then remove from heat.

8. Add coriander leaves then serve spiced rice alongside carrot and cumin salad.

10. Cured Pollock with dill cream and radish salad

Nutritional Value: Calories 463, Fat 37, protein 27 g, Net carbs 5g.

Preparation time – 20 mins cooking time –25 mins

Servings – 4

Ingredients

- Fennel seeds – 100g

- Chopped small pack dill – 1

- Skinless Pollock fillet – 400g

- Rapeseed oil – 500ml

- Golden caster sugar – 100g

- Coarse salt – 100g

For the dill cream

- Full fat cream – 140g

- Cayenne pepper to season

- Chopped small pack dill – ½

- Finely grated zest lemon – 1

For radish salad

- Radishes – 300g

- Taramasalata – 1 tablespoon

- Lemon juice – ½

- Snipped pack chives – ½

- Smoked paprika – ½ teaspoon

Instructions

1. In a large bowl, mix together salt, sugar, dill and fennel seeds then use a cling film to line a large dish.

2. Place Pollock fillet in the bowl then add the remaining salt mix on top. Spread the cling film on top then completely cover the fish. Place it in the fridge as you give it time to cure overnight or for about 8 hours.

3. The fish will then become firm and with a salty flavor. You can then wash the salt off as you place it in a large dish then allow to soak in cold water for about 30 minutes.

4. Drain the water from the fish; you can use kitchen paper to dry it up.

5. Get the oven heated to 150C then place the fish in a roasting tin. Pour rapeseed oil over the fish then cover with a sheet of foil as you seal around the edges. Allow it to cook for about 25 minutes.

6. Remove from the oven then set aside at room temperature.

7. Wash the radishes then cut in half then in a bowl whisk together taramasalata and lemon juice.

8. Remove Pollock then drain excess oil as you flake it on a large plate. Add cooking oil to taramasalata then whisk together.

9. Add radishes, smoked paprika and chives to the dressing then fold it together as you ensure the radishes are well coated.

10. Serve the fish with dill and the radish salad. You can enjoy it with toasted bread.

11. Cloud Bread

Nutritional Value: Calories 59, Fat 5, protein 3 g, Net carbs 0.2g.

Preparation time – 10 mins cooking time –20mins

Servings – 8 pieces

Ingredients

- Oil or butter (for greasing)

- Eggs – 4

- Cream cheese – 50g

- Nigella seeds – ½ teaspoon

Instructions

1. Get the oven heated to 150C

2. Have the baking sheets lined with baking paper as you grease with oil or butter.

3. Whisk egg whites together in a large bowl then in another bowl place the egg yolks, cream of tartar and cream cheese then whisk all together until smooth.

4. Fold the egg whites into yolk mixture then fold in nigella seeds as you also season with pepper and salt.

5. On the prepared baking sheets dollop the mixture then allow to bake for about 20 minutes or until craggy at the top or lightly golden.

6. Allow to cool then carefully remove from the paper.

7. Serve and enjoy

12. Greek salad omelet

Nutritional Value: Calories 371, Fat 28, protein 24g, Net carbs 5g.

Preparation time – 10 mins cooking time –10mins

Servings – 4

Ingredients

- Eggs – 10

- Chopped parsley leaves (handful)

- Olive oil – 2 tablespoons

- Large red onion - 1

- Chopped tomatoes – 3

- Black olives (handful)

- Crumbled feta cheese – 100g

Instructions

1. Have the grill heated to high the in a large bowl whisk the eggs and add chopped parsley, salt and pepper.

2. In non-stick frying pan heat oil then add onion wedges and fry over high heat for about 4 minutes.

3. Add in tomatoes and olive then cook for 2 minutes or until the tomatoes become soft.

4. Reduce the heat to medium then add eggs and allow to cook for 2 minutes.

5. Scatter the eggs over feta then grill for 6 minutes or until the omelet gets golden and puffed up.

6. Cut into wedges then serve and enjoy.

Chapter 8

Ketogenic Snacks/Desserts Recipes

1. Low carb cheesecake

Nutritional Value: Calories 415 , Fat 38, protein 11g, Net carbs 3g.

Preparation time – 12 mins cooking time –1.30mins

Servings – 12 slices

Ingredients

Crust

- Almonds – ½ cup

- Pecans – ½ cup

- Butter – 6 tablespoons

- Protein powder – 1 scoop

- Cinnamon – ½ tablespoon

- Liquid stevia – 10 drops

- Salt

Cheesecake

- Cream Cheese – 32 oz

- Erythritol – 2/3 cup

- Liquid stevia – 20 drops

- Large eggs – 4

- Vanilla Extract – 2 tablespoons

- Fresh lemon juice

- Sour cream – ½ cup

- Himalayan salt – ½ teaspoon

Instructions

1. Heat the oven to 3250F

2. To make the crust; on a clean baking sheet toast pecans and almonds then bake for 10 minutes. Toss once halfway to ensure both sides are well toasted. Remove as you allow the oven to stay on.

3. Once toasted, place them into a food processor with other crust ingredients then blend.

4. Use your fingers to press the crust then bake for 10 minutes or until it turns golden. Allow the crust to cool once cooked before adding cheesecake batter.

5. To prepare cheesecake batter, mix together cream cheese, stevia, and erythritol then process with an electric hand mixer for a smooth and soft mixture.

6. Add one egg at a time as you incorporate each into the mixture. Add lemon juice, vanilla extract, and salt.

7. Add sour cream then stir until well combined.

8. Pour in the cheesecake batter as you smooth the top with a spatula. In a spring form pan pour hot water until halfway up.

9. Transfer into the oven the roasting pan alongside the spring form pan then bake for one hour.

10. Once the cake has baked, turn off the oven and leave the doo open for the cake to cool off. Let the cake stay for about an hour before covering and refrigerating.

11. Top the cake with your preferred toppings then enjoy.

2. Caramel Nut Clusters

Nutritional Value: Calories 90, Fat 8, protein 1, Net carbs 1.5g.

Preparation time – 25mins cooking time –10mins

Servings – 9 clusters

Ingredients

Base

- Pecans – 9

- Macadamias – 20

- Caramel candies – 9 (sugar-free)

- Coarse sea salt – 1 tablespoon

Chocolate Ganache

- Heavy cream – 3 tablespoons

- Dark chocolate – 40g

- Vanilla Extract – ¼ teaspoon

Instructions

1. Get the oven preheated to 320F

2. Get the baking sheet lined with parchment paper. Arrange the pecans then add macadamia nuts close to them.

3. Place caramel candy on each pile then transfer carefully to the oven. Let it bake for 10 minutes then allow to cool.

4. To make chocolate ganache, place a small pot over low heat then heat the cream until it gets bubbly. Add dark chocolate and allow it to melt as you stir gently. Add vanilla extract to the mixture and then stir to combine.

5. Once the chocolate is silky and smooth, add 1 teaspoon of chocolate to the pile of nuts then sprinkle sea salt onto the candies when the chocolate is still wet.

6. Refrigerate for an hour then enjoy.

3.   Low Carb Peanut Butter Cookies

Nutritional Value: Calories 105 , Fat 9, protein 4g, Net carbs 2g.

Preparation time – 10 mins cooking time –10mins

Servings – 15

Ingredients

- Peanut butter – 1 cup

- Erythritol – ½ cup

- Egg – 1

Instructions

1. Get the oven preheated to 350F

2. Gather all the ingredients then place granulated erythritol into a blender then blend for a few seconds.

3. Combine the powdered erythritol. Peanut butter and the egg into a bowl then mix well.

4. Roll the cookie into balls then place them on a baking sheet lined with parchment then bake for 15 minutes until the cookies turn darker.

5. Allow the cookies to cool then enjoy with a glass of nut milk.

4. Salted Caramel Custard

Nutritional Value: Calories 273, Fat 27g protein 9g, Net carbs 1.5g.

Preparation time – 10 mins cooking time –10mins

Servings – 2

Ingredients

Custard

- Eggs – 2

- Softened cream cheese – 2 oz

- Water - 1 cup

- Granulated sugar substitute

- Caramel extract – 1.5 tablespoon

Caramel Sauce

- Salted butter – 2 tablespoon

- Granulated sugar substitute - 2 tablespoon

- Caramel extract

Instructions

1. Get the oven preheated to 3250F

2. Combine all the custard ingredients in a blender then blend until smooth.

3. Pour into two bowls then place on a cookie sheet and into the oven. Pour hot water into the cookie sheets up to halfway the sides of the bowls.

4. Bake for about 30 minutes then remove and allow to chill for

about one hour before you serve.

5. To prepare the sauce: Melt the butter, caramel flavoring, and sweetener then microwave for about 30 seconds or until well blended.

6. Divide into half then pour onto the custards before serving.

7. Serve and enjoy

5. Walnut Keto Fudge

Nutritional Value: Calories 134, Fat 14.1, protein 1.8g, Net carbs 2.2g.

Preparation time – 10mins cooking time –10mins

Servings – 12 pcs

Ingredients

- Softened butter – 120g

- Softened cream cheese 120g

- Dark cocoa powder – 3 tablespoons

- Granulated sweetener – 2 tablespoons

- Vanilla – 1 tablespoon

- Walnut – 40g

Instructions

1. Mix together softened butter with cream cheese until well combined without lumps.

2. Add cocoa, vanilla and sweetener then mix thoroughly

3. Add walnuts and mix gently

4. Place the mixture into a lined dish then put into the fridge.

5. Slice then serve and enjoy.

6.   Coconut Cream with Berries

Nutritional Value: Fat 89%, protein 4%g, Net carbs 6%g.

Preparation time – cooking time –2mins

Servings – 1

Ingredients

- Coconut cream - 6 ¾ tablespoons

- Fresh strawberries – 2/3 oz

- Vanilla extract – 1 pinch

Instructions

1. Mix all the ingredients together then blend.

2. Add 1 tablespoon of coconut oil for increased fat ratio.

7.   Berries and whipped Cream

Nutritional Value: Fat 88%, protein 4%, Net carbs 7%.

Preparation time – 15mins cooking time

Servings – 2

Ingredients

- Fresh raspberries, strawberries or blueberries – 1 cup

- Heavy whipping cream – 2/3 cup

- Vanilla extract – ¼ cup

Instructions

1. If the berries are frozen then allow them to come to room temperature.

2. Whip the cream until fluffy with soft peaks. The cream should not be too firm or grainy.

3. Add vanilla extract then serve immediately alongside the berries.

4. Serve and enjoy

8. Pumpkin Pecan Tart

Nutritional Value: Calories 530, Fat 45, protein 19g, Net carbs 9g.

Preparation time – 30mins cooking time –30mins

Servings – 2

Ingredients

- Almond flour – ½ cup

- Melted butter – 2 tablespoons

- Cinnamon – 1 tablespoon

- Salt

Filling

- Ricotta cheese – ½ cup

- Pumpkin puree – ½ cup

- Cinnamon – 1 tablespoon

- Vanilla extract – ½ tablespoon

- Salt

- Erythritol – 2 tablespoon

- Egg – 1

Topping

- Pecans – 16

- Sugar-free maple syrup

Instructions

1. Get the oven preheated to 350F

2. Combine all the ingredients for the crust into a bowl then mix thoroughly.

3. Press the mixture into two tarts then give them time to cool.

4. For the filling combine the pumpkin puree, ricotta cheese, and the egg then add the sweetener, flavorings and salt.

5. Mix all together until well combined.

6. Once the crusts have cooled, pour the fillings then place on a baking sheet and allow to bake for 20 minutes.

7. Remove once the time is up then add pecans on top. Return to the oven then allow to bake for 10 more minutes.

8. Remove from the oven once baked then allow to cool slightly.

9. Drizzle with the maple syrup and some cream. Enjoy

9. Sugar-Free Chocolate Chips

Nutritional Value: Calories 28, Fat 3, protein 0.2g, Net carbs 0.1g.

Preparation time – 20mins cooking time –

Servings – 2

Ingredients

- Butter – 4 tablespoons

- Heavy cream – 1 tablespoon

- Powdered erythritol – 3 tablespoon

- Vanilla extract – ¼ teaspoon

- Salt

Instructions

1. Melt butter and the unsweetened bakers chocolate then stir well.

2. Add heavy cream and the powdered erythritol then stir.

3. Add vanilla and salt then stir.

4. Crack sea salt into the mold then pour chocolate batter

5. Shake it up for the chocolate to spread well to the corners.

6. Freeze the chocolate for about an hour.

7. Pour chocolate bar batter into silicone pot holder.

8. Use a spatula to spread into each cavity

9. Place into the freezer then let it freeze for about 2 hours

10. Once frozen, twist the molds to allow the chocolate chips to

pop out onto a plate.

11. Enjoy the chocolate chips.

10. Basic Oopsie Rolls

Nutritional Value: Calories 45, Fat 4, protein 2g, Net carbs 0g.

Preparation time – 20mins cooking time –35mins

Servings – 12 pcs

Ingredients

- Large eggs – 3

- Cream cheese - 3 oz

- Cream of tartar – 1/8 teaspoon

- Salt

Instructions

1. Get the oven preheated to 300F

2. Separate the eggs yolks from whites then set in different bowls.

3. Beat the egg whites until bubbly

4. Add cream of tartar then whisk together.

5. In the bowl with egg yolk, add cream cheese and salt.

6. Whisk together until pale yellow.

7. Gently fold together the cream cheese mixture into the egg whites

8. Line cookie sheet with parchment paper then spray oil to grease it.

9. Dollop the oopsie roll batter onto the cookie sheet then place in the oven and bake for about 40 minutes or until the rolls become firm and golden.

10. Allow to cool then serve and enjoy.

Chapter 9

Tips to help you succeed at the Ketogenic Diet

If you are to succeed with the ketogenic diet then there are tips that you need to follow:

1. Calorie Intake and the Ketogenic Diet

The counting of calories can be of great help especially in providing one with a rough idea on the quantity of carbs, fat, and proteins that can be taken on a given day. As much as you don't have to strictly count calories whenever you are purchasing food, it's important that you have some idea on the amount of calories that you should be taking in a given day if you are to realize weight loss and other benefits that are associated with ketogenic diet. In fact, with a ketogenic diet, you will realize that you eat less food yet feel more satisfied most of the times which then translates to less intake of calories.

If you stick to the given ratio of 5% carbs, 25% proteins and 75% fats, then you will see that all you have to do is to focus on the ratios and not amounts of calories and you will be assured of success with the ketogenic diet.

2. Hydration and the Ketogenic Diet

Keeping your body hydrated is a very important factor when you are on a ketogenic diet. Since your body gets to efficiently burn fat, you will no longer feel tired or irritable as you may have been when you were on a high carb diet. However, your body loses more water in the process which demands that you increase your water intake to stay hydrated. Drinking more water will, therefore, result in more success with the keto diet.

3. The Ketogenic Diet and Your Budget

Eating healthy is generally more expensive when compared to eating the highly processed foods that may seem cheap yet have been proven to be the cause of most of the health problems that many people face today. Many people shy away from a ketogenic diet because they assume it's more expensive than the traditional diet. But, you will realize that when you let go of the highly processed foods like cookies, chips, cakes, noodles, grains, and rice, you will have more than enough to spend on a ketogenic diet.

There are still a few techniques that you can take advantage of to ensure that you have success with the diet. For example, you can engage in the following:

- Purchasing foods in bulk so that you don't keep going to the grocery store regularly.

- Consider what you are buying before spending the money instead of impulse buying.

- You can look out for deals on foods where you get to buy at discount prices.

- You can freeze foods in bulk so that you save on energy costs as you also avoid wastage of food.

- You can make use of coupons. Saving a few dollars here and there can be valuable in the long run.

4.   Traveling While Eating Keto

Many people find it challenging to stick to a keto diet, especially when they are traveling. However, it's possible to stick to your keto diet even when traveling. With proper preparation and planning, you can find out about places where you can get to eat your preferred food before traveling. Instead of opting to eat foods provided by the hotel, attempt to find a room with a kitchen so you may cook your meals. When dining out, focus on cheese, vegetables, and meat when you are uncertain of what to eat. Stay away from soft drinks and beer.

5.   Fast Food Choices and Keto

There are people who shy away from a ketogenic diet just because they feel they have limited choices for fast foods while dieting. When it comes to fast foods, remember to stick to the following:

1. Ensure that you stick to cheese, meat, and vegetables. Look out for the excess sugar and carbs that are normally stuffed in fast food so that you don't end up compromising your dieting process.

2. Avoid buns or breads. Remember, it's made from the grains which are high in carbs. Opt for the extras like bacon or avocado.

3. If you are to go for salads, then be on the lookout for the ingredients as some of the vegetables are known to have high levels of carbohydrates.

4. Watch out for the condiments as some may be filled with sugar. Try to avoid consuming anything that can throw you out of

ketosis.

5. Look out for the nutrition information, especially if you are ordering online so that you are sure of the composition of the foods.

6. Working out on a Ketogenic Diet

You can still be on a ketogenic diet and engage in exercises. However, you should ensure that you eat sufficient protein for that lean body mass. You can also increase your calorie intake as it's not easy to build muscles without increasing intake of calories. Training correctly is also vital if you are to hypertrophy in the muscles. Consider consuming carbohydrates 30 minutes before your routine as a way to supplement your energy levels, especially for high-intensity workouts. Look at the targeted ketogenic diet variation in chapter 1.

7. Fasting and Ketosis

Fasting can be of great benefit especially if you are shifting from high carb diet to a ketogenic diet. As you engage in fasting, your body becomes deficient of glucose which then enables it to adapt much faster to burning fat for fuel. However, it's important that you strictly follow the ratio so that you don't mess the process of ketosis once your body has adapted to it. Fasting is recommended for about 2-4 days, especially during the initial stages as extending longer may put your body into a state of starvation which may not be healthy.

Conclusion

Congratulations and thank you for investing in this book and reading it all through. Keto Diet: The Ultimate Guide to Everything Keto is a book that has shared, in detail, all that the ketogenic diet entails and gives comprehensive insights regarding the ketogenic diet.

If you intend to reap the numerous benefits shared in this book, then the best way to do so is by putting what you have read into practice. From understanding what the ketogenic diet is, the numerous benefits associated with the diet, the process of the body shifting from burning glucose to burning fat, to the nutritious ketogenic recipes that have been shared in the book. All that you have read in this book has the potential of helping you in realizing success with the ketogenic diet.

Now implement what you have read and if you're not certain about an area, then the best thing to do is to go through it again even as you verify with other sources. I know that you have found the book to be valuable and all that I have is a request, please go ahead and leave a review for the book now that you have read it through.

Thank you and enjoy your keto diet journey.

Don't Forget to Download Your FREE 25 Ketogenic Diet Dessert Recipes

Get these 25 additional dessert recipes that will make it seem like it's cheat day!

http://dibblypublishing.com/free-25ketodessertrecipes/

Other Books Published by Dibbly Publishing

Affirmations: Powerful Affirmations to Empower the Subconscious Mind to Achieve Anything

By: Garry Hudson

Self-Discipline: A How to Guide on Overcoming Laziness and Conquering Procrastination

By: Spence Adams

Habits: How to Implement Essential Habits to Improve Productivity, Success, and Wealth

By: Spence Adams

Made in the USA
San Bernardino, CA
21 November 2017